BE FIT! OR BE DAMNED!

PERCY WELLS CERUTTY

Olympic Coach — Australia
10 January 1895 – 14 August 1975

A Classic Revival from

www.pmabooks.com

This book first published in 1967
by Pelham Books Ltd, London, WC1

This edition published 2014 by
PMA Books, Classic Revival Series
Brisbane, Australia
with the kind permission
of the Percy Cerutty Estate
©Percy Cerutty 1967

Copyright of all pictures belongs to the author

A Classic Revival from

www.pmabooks.com

PO Box 5197, Manly Qld 4179 AUSTRALIA
Tel + 61 488 224 929 * m. 0488 224 929
PUBLISHING DIRECTOR: Judy Hinz
email judyhinz@pmabooks.com
0411 592 386

CONTENTS

FOREWORD   10

PUBLISHER'S FOREWORD AND DISCLAIMER   11

PREFACE   13

INTRODUCTION   20

CHAPTER ONE   24
What man is: how long on Earth: the time scale: how he lived for countless centuries: caves: wild animals and stress: exercise: food.

CHAPTER TWO   33
Statistics: longevity: recent high averages of life expectancy due to: expectancy in animals as against man.

CHAPTER THREE   40
The physiology of Man: the heart, lungs, liver and kidneys.

CHAPTER FOUR   53
The brain; mind; illusions; disillusionments and frustrations.

CHAPTER FIVE   60
Life as a challenge: repressing emotion and the blood pressure: stress and ulcers.

CHAPTER SIX   69
The chief destroyers: de-natured foods: nicotine, not worry: alcohol, not over-work: barbiturates (sleeping pills, sedatives – even aspirin, and the like): gambling a cause of stress

CHAPTER SEVEN 77
A sound basic philosophy is necessary: the need to recognise what life is: realism and religion: self reliance and saviours: wealth: privileges: investments: even pensions – can disappear: fitness can always be there.

CHAPTER EIGHT 89
The heart as the key: diet as the chief means: something on the elements of our foods: the importance of vitamins and trace elements.

CHAPTER NINE 97
Fats: milk: starches: sugars: salt: vitamins: vegetarianism: raw foods: fluids.

CHAPTER TEN 108
Certain ideas, axioms and principles need to be understood, and adopted. These factors apply to hunger, weight, and over-feeding.

CHAPTER ELEVEN 113
On exercise: why it is essential to exercise: man's main weakness: the two chief exercises: the degree of exertion in walking and running.

CHAPTER TWELVE 121
Still on exercise: after energetic walking, or steady running, the next important exercises are those that strengthen, and maintain the tone of the back and abdominal muscles

CHAPTER THIRTEEN 129
Dead-Lifting: The Basic and Best Exercise, and most natural of all Exercises using apparatus.

CHAPTER FOURTEEN 137
If you grow to love the barbell – here are some more exercises.

CHAPTER FIFTEEN — 147
Some measure-rods: criteria and means of determining the degree of fitness, together with the indications and warnings that precede unfitness and early or eventual demise short of what might have been.

CHAPTER SIXTEEN — 153
A daily exercise schedule for the busy man prepared to devote no more than 15 minutes per day to his fitness.

CHAPTER SEVENTEEN — 161
A daily exercise schedule for the man prepared to devote 30 minutes per day to his fitness and physical well-being.

CHAPTER EIGHTEEN — 168
On Ageing.

CHAPTER NINETEEN — 172
Human elimination.

CHAPTER TWENTY — 176
The large city destroys: the country gives life.

CHAPTER TWENTY ONE — 179
In conclusion, and to repeat.

SOME CONCLUSIONS — 181
APPENDIX ONE: mostly philosophic

APPENDIX TWO 'IF' (with apologies to Rudyard Kipling)

APPENDIX THREE: a recapitulation of the book in axiomatic form

APPENDIX FOUR: suggestions for dietary

Illustrations

ILLUSTRATION 1   17
Stretching the arms and body upwards

ILLUSTRATION 2   17
Making an effort to touch the toes

ILLUSTRATION 3   17
Stretching the arms and twisting the body while sitting

ILLUSTRATION 4   18
Posture when walking

ILLUSTRATION 5   18
Moving from a walk into a run

ILLUSTRATION 6   27
Another part of a stride in running

ILLUSTRATION 7   27
Another part of a stride

ILLUSTRATION 8   28
The Sit-up exercise

ILLUSTRATION 9	**28**
The finish position of the sit-up	
ILLUSTRATION 10	**43**
The press-up	
ILLUSTRATION 11	**43**
The finish of the press-up	
ILLUSTRATION 12	**44**
The prone-press	
ILLUSTRATION 13	**44**
The finish of the prone-press	
ILLUSTRATION 14	**63**
Correct position and angle of the body	
ILLUSTRATION 15	**63**
The finish of the dead-lift	
ILLUSTRATION 16	**63**
Side view of the finish of the dead-lift	
ILLUSTRATION 17	**64**
The dead-lift	
ILLUSTRATION 18	**64**
The dead-lift performed in the correct way	
ILLUSTRATION 19	**64**
The weight about to leave the ground	

ILLUSTRATION 20	81
The rowing motion	

ILLUSTRATION 21	82
The cheat curl	

ILLUSTRATION 22	82
Finishing the cheat curl	

ILLUSTRATION 23	86
The author commencing a cheat curl	

ILLUSTRATION 24	86
Finish of the cheat curl	

ILLUSTRATION 25	87
Commencing a one-arm press	

ILLUSTRATION 26	87
Movement just before the completion of the upward throw	

ILLUSTRATION 27	104
Start of the one-handed swing	

ILLUSTRATION 28	104
Completion of the one-handed swing	

ILLUSTRATION 29	105
The bench-press	

ILLUSTRATION 30	105
The bench-press completed	

ILLUSTRATION 31	125
The sit-up using an inclined board	

ILLUSTRATION 32	125
The completion of the sit-up on the inclined board	

ILLUSTRATION 33	126
Chin on the horizontal bar	

ILLUSTRATION 34	126
The author, aged 72	

ILLUSTRATION 35	142
The author leaving the sea with a number of runners – midwinter	

ILLUSTRATION 36	142
The author running at 70 years of age	

ILLUSTRATION 37	143
The author, body weight, 130 lb., lifting a lad weighing 14 stone	

ILLUSTRATION 38	157
The author running the sand hill at Portsea (Australia) with his pupil Herb Elliott	

ILLUSTRATION 39	158
The author with his publisher William Luscombe and a newspaper editor in Tokyo. Olympic Games, 1964	

ILLUSTRATION 40	158
The author with his stepdaughter Elaine	

Foreword

This book is addressed to the above-average intelligent, successful, and older man.

It was written to supply the essential knowledge that all men should have, and especially for the man who has not had the time, or possibly, the inclination, to study extensively the findings of the Scientists and the Medical Profession, the literature of which, today, is most extensive.

Nor does the reader have to grapple with the scientific and medical phraseology and nomenclature, just as he does not have to worry through the findings of the health and fitness experts, the Psychiatrists, even the Philosophers and Theologians.

Be Fit! Or Be Damned! encompasses all the findings in simple language, with perhaps, some of the reasons, and in a form that the reader can quickly and readily comprehend.

There can be only one hope: that the reader will find the subject matter interesting, convincing, and that he will act upon it.

Publisher's Foreword and Disclaimer

This book was written in the 1960s and is republished here without alteration. Some of the concepts, ideas and scientific knowledge expressed by the author Percy Cerutty were his opinions and observations set against the background of knowledge at the time of writing.

Some readers may consider some of the statements to be bordering on the outrageous but it is well to remember that Percy Cerutty was not only a man ahead of his time but also a man of very firm opinions. I encourage you to read the book with this thought very firmly in your mind.

The underlying message is a positive one and it is up to the well informed reader to implement any of Percy Cerutty's ideas through the filter of modern knowledge.

A word of caution too – you should always consult with your medical professionals before undertaking strenuous and unusual exercise.

I'd like to point out to readers also that his reference to the Australian Aborigines hunting in the Great Sandy Desert, seemingly living the same existence they have for thousands of years and untouched by 'civilised' society, is something that has been consigned to history. I would acknowledge that there are any number of difficult issues surrounding Australia's first people and their attempts to bridge the gulf between their traditional society and the modern society introduced by European settlement in

1788 but to my knowledge none remain in their pre-1788 existence.

I trained at Percy Cerutty's Portsea camp in the Christmas vacation period of 1964-65. I was a schoolboy athlete, who had shown some promise over the middle distances. I wasn't destined to become a champion athlete but nevertheless Percy Cerutty had a significant impact on my life.

I invite you to read his book and take from it the important lessons he was imparting to his aspiring athletes back in the 1960s.

Peter Masters
Director
PMA Books

Preface

> *'It is not merely that you are alive but how much alive you are that is important.'*

Any book on health and fitness must start with what man is – his physical body, the nature of his mind, and the needs of both.

Man, under the conditions of civilization, if he is to enjoy a fit survival, must have some knowledge of his pre-historic origins: the construction of his body: the skeleton, muscles and organs, and the strengths and weaknesses of the various parts.

It is one of the astonishing facts of modern life that a man will spend many years in fitting himself to earn a livelihood, but spends little or no time in discovering what he is as a machine that does the earning.

Because he may enjoy normally good health in his early manhood, he does not consider it necessary to understand, not only what he is – his nature, but the remarkably complicated piece of machinery his body actually is. Therefore, he acts, thinks and lives, as if his body was something detached from him as a person: something that can be ignored as to its vital needs and treatment.

He imagines, if he thinks about it at all, that his mind (brain) is everything: that his appetites are normal, or that he can abuse, neglect or poison his body with impunity: just as if it was something separate from his mind, and his personality.

When, after some years of neglect, or actual abuse, he finds he has one of the many diseases common in modern Society, he attributes the fact to 'bad luck'. He seldom realises that his coronary, his high blood pressure, his cirrhosis, his rheumatism, mostly called fibrositis today, even his tumours and cancers, are all preventable, NOT by drugs, but by understanding his bodily organism, caring for it and nourishing it, and exercising it, as he is customarily prepared to do for his race-horse, even his automobile, in the sense of proper care and maintenance.

In a word, man pays considerably more intelligent attention to his live-stock, and upon his machinery, than ever he does upon his most personal machine, his own body.

Furthermore, he is inclined to the idea, if he ever thinks about it at all, that the way he lives, the foods he eats, is the way his ancestors lived and ate. He seldom reflects upon the way man evolved: the way he lived for countless millenniums of time, and how different these are to the way he lives today.

He seriously believes that his appetite for food, good, bad or indifferent, is a reliable guide. Indeed, he has a rather juvenile attitude to most things because of his lack of knowledge as to his body and its needs. He even believes that his brain produces for him all the right answers, whatever his problem may be.

He, mankind in general, never appears to realise that the brain as we know it, and distinct from its instinctive processes, is a relatively recent addition to man, that only a few thousand years ago man did not use his brain as modern man does simply because primitive society did not contain in itself any reasons for such brain development, education, or use: that it was a relatively un-evolved and dormant organ.

It would appear to be a truism that man, mostly, only 'thinks he thinks': that his decisions and actions based in brain-work can only be right as he has full and true knowledge, no matter what it may be he thinks about.

Actually, the brain of mankind, is nothing more than a most remarkable computer. It digests what is fed into it by education and experience, and, together with inherent environmental factors, produces the 'answers' accordingly. Left in a state of complete lack of education, as is the case, with idiocy, or complete isolation, other than instinctive reactions, the brain, of itself, can produce little or nothing.

Whatever man thinks, or his brain produces in answers, feed another set of 'facts', or experiences, into his brain and it will produce an entirely different set of answers.

It now appears evident that civilised man, by virtue of his brain, and his belief in it as to the rightness of his way of life, has departed from the natural needs of his body and its functions, even to losing the capacity for reasonably healthy survival.

This is more obvious when we study the statistics as they apply to the number and lethal qualities of the diseases that assail mankind, and the poor level of health of many, even before reaching maturity. Add to this the premature demise of the many, and the increasing number requiring some form of psychiatric treatment, the incidence of alcoholism and drug-taking, and the picture is neither pleasant nor reassuring.

Man, as an organism, and a highly evolved organism or creature, carries within himself the means of resistance to many of the breakdowns, and much of the disease, that assails him. But, powerful as these resistances are in the beginning, once the organism has been broken down by the abuse of it, or by ignorant ill-treatment, the inevitable collapse is often speedy, as it is always eventually certain.

There is no substitution for a heart that has ceased to beat: for a liver so diseased that it cannot function: for kidneys that can no longer filter. All these, and some others, spelled – death, and only too often, preventable death.

This, then, is the reason for this book. It is an attempt to make it clear, and beyond reasonable doubt, that with knowledge, elementary as it may be, and living within the capacity of the bodily functions, man may reasonably be expected to control, and prolong his life, much more than the many ever could realise.

The Rules are simple, but adamant. Self-discipline is an essential to this well-being: the Key is – knowledge. This book, in simple, every-day language, purports to place this knowledge before you. It is YOU, the Reader, who must apply it.

EN AVANT!

Summary of Preface: and to Repeat:

Man needs knowledge of what he is: his origins: the construction of his body: knowledge as to his muscles and organs.

Man spends years on learning how to earn: little or no time on how to live.

Man acts and thinks detached from a consideration as to the needs of his body as a complicated piece of machinery, robust withal.

Man imagines the Brain to be all: infallible: that his appetites are normal: mostly, he is indifferent to the needs of his body, other than indulgences.

Man seldom realises that the diseases he is mostly heir to are avoidable.

Man believes, if he thinks about it at all, that the way he lives, what he eats, is the way man always lived and ate.

Man believes his appetite for food is a reliable guide. Actually, his general knowledge about himself and his needs are juvenile, due to ignorance. He believes his brain can produce all the right answers for him. It cannot.

PREFACE

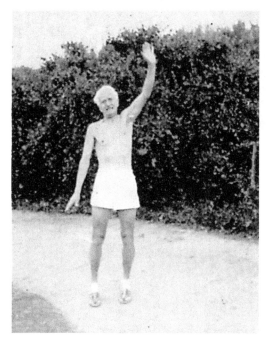

Stretching Exercises: Stretching the arms and body upwards. Both arms should be stretched up alternately until a feeling of pain is experienced. This exercise is essential to counter the normal constriction, the shortening of the muscles, the shrinkage that is experienced with age, the sinking to the ground of the body-bulk and which shortens the stature.

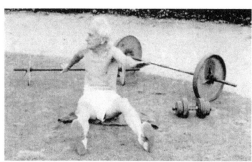

Stretching the arms and twisting the body whilst sitting. An essential exercise to maintain body fluidity, i.e. to resist the onslaught of stiffness of the joints and lack of flexibility.

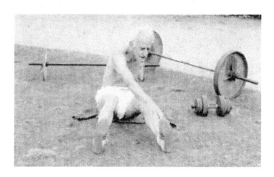

Another form of stretching where the effort is made to touch the toes with the opposite hand. The Stretching Exercises can be done standing. Any form of stretching is good. Note: Animals, of which the easiest to observe are the domestic cat and dog, always stretch after resting.

PREFACE

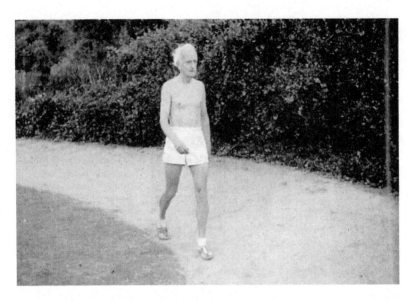

Posture when walking. Note the in-toeing of the foot, and the suggestion of complete bodily relaxation.

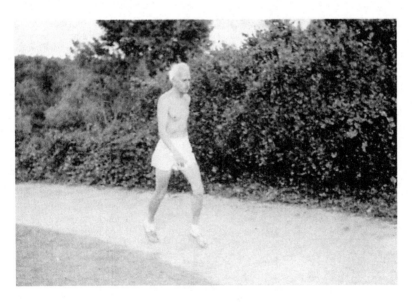

Moving from a walk into a run. Note that the arms remain low and have not been lifted as is so customarily, but wrongly, seen

PREFACE

Man, mostly, only 'thinks' he thinks. The brain is mostly a computer, producing answers as information is fed into it. Of itself, without facts fed in, the brain can produce nothing. Feed in one set off acts and we get one answer. Feed in another set and the answer will be different.

Man believes his way of life, because he experiences it, must be good: correct: the total answer.

His diseases and, often early demise proves something is not right with his way of life.

Man carries within himself much resistance to bodily breakdown, but once ignorance and abuse has broken his natural resistances down the inevitable collapse is often rapid.

There is no substitute for diseased, faulty, or broken-down hearts, livers, lungs and kidneys.

This book suggests that, when he acquires the simple knowledge he needs, and acts upon it, he can prolong his life, considerably, and happily.

The Rules to do this are simple, but self-discipline is essential. The key is knowledge. This book supplies the knowledge. YOU, the Reader, must apply it.

Introduction

The high incidence of death from diseases of the circulatory system, that is the heart, the arteries, and the organs directly associated with the blood, and its purity, viz.: mainly, the liver and kidneys, as well as the lethal strokes due to artery lesion in the brain, and being more than half the causes of death in most, if not all, civilised countries: these, together with Carcinoma (cancer in its many forms and organ incidence) account for, perhaps, 90 per cent of all deaths: Yet all these diseases are preventable.

In Australia, for 1963, the total deaths from all causes was 98,000 in round figures. These deaths included child diseases, tuberculosis, venereal, cancer, accidents of all kinds, and the many diseases of the circulatory system.

Of all these causes, the diseases that could be traced directly, or indirectly, to a failure of some part of the circulatory system accounted for no less than 84,000.

This, then, is the reason for this book.

The Author will claim that he had no special franchise or right to live. Indeed, in childhood, there was every reason why he should have died. But, like the proverbial cat, he would appear to have had nine lives. It was the 'instinct to survive' born, or later developed, that turned the scale in his favour.

This book, then, is written so that you, the reader, can turn the scale, if you would turn it, in your favour. Otherwise it is to leave it to luck, your inheritance of vitality, perhaps instinctive intelligence. But it is a truism that knowledge is power: destiny can be converted to our purposes, and that we can control our sojourn, if not our entry into this world, at least our passage through it, and our ultimate and final demise much more than most people appear to realise.

So we will set out clearly and without ambiguity, in non-technical language, just what man is: what he needs for his well-being and survival: and the effect modern civilization has upon him: its lethal qualities, and the steps he must take if – he is to survive.

And survival does not imply the biblical three score years and ten; when man should have achieved, if he ever is to achieve it, reality; meaning, understanding what this world is: what this life is: his part in it: wisdom and a patriarchal position.

Man should, and could, having achieved reality and the 'allotted span', find that he does not die, but enjoys his heritage, and this heritage should be, could be, another 'span' of half a century, or a second span of three score years and ten.

Bluntly, and it has been stated by many authorities, man should live, if he but knew how, for 120 years to 150 years, possibly longer. And this does not mean 'limp' along senile, aged, and ineffective, but using his accumulated experience, wisdom and knowledge, in the service of mankind: useful, active, vigorous, and virile, as he well may be, and could be, shall we say – should be.

If needs must be recognised that age is not measured only by solar time – days, months and years. Agedness can be advanced, or retarded, as we understand the means for so-doing. Because most men, almost all men, know little of these things, preoccupied as they mostly are, in business, and the affairs of the World, in no way is a negation of his statement, as it in no way exonerates man from the charge of being ignorant, and through ignorance, foolish or self-destructive.

This book, then, is dedicated to the man (and woman) who has a desire to live – intelligently, usefully, happily, and fully – far beyond the customary expectancy, which is – NOT 70! even, but only too often, merely some time in the forties, if lucky in the fifties, or in the sixties with a 'heart', a cancer, or, at the best, a lack-luster life – little or no activity: little art: little music: little zest, perhaps no women: little or nothing – worth living for!

No wonder Shakespeare said 'The fault, dear Brutus, is not in our stars, but in ourselves, that we are underlings', and to paraphrase this, I say: We can make of ourselves what we may make, that the solution, or key, to our problems lie within us: that the rewards are in exact proportion as we are prepared to learn: to think: to act.

No sensible man believes in luck as a substitution for work, or knowledge. The day is past, if it ever existed, when it was sensible to say, 'Why worry! Tomorrow we may all be dead', or, 'I've been lucky so far, why should I worry'.

Inexorable statistics face us. Nature has no favourites. Those born stronger, more resistant than the many may escape, or postpone, the moment of truth. Do not be deceived by that story of the one in a thousand, or the one in a million, who did, or was said to do, all the things that ordinarily kill people, but he seemed to have a charmed life.

Sensible people take no such risks: invite no such chances: and believe in no such fables. After all, discretion IS the better part of valour: and a wise man takes no unnecessary risks. Finally, as the advertisement has it – 'Death is so permanent'.

Summary to the Introduction

Probably 90 per cent of all deaths are due to a breakdown somewhere of the circulatory system. This involves the Heart, Liver, Kidney and Lungs, plus Cancer, but which whilst not part of the circulatory system is involved in it.

INTRODUCTION

The author had no special right to live. Sickness and the desire to survive forced him to experiment and learn. He would attempt to pass his knowledge on to you, as the reader, that you may have the information that tends to exclude luck, or favourable inherited factors, that you may or may not have, as the decisive factors.

With knowledge all things are possible. Man can control his destiny. Accurate knowledge provides the means to avoid the lethal factors in modern life. Unlimited survival: not merely three score years and ten. Attaining some comprehension of reality man can, conceivably, add another three score years and ten, to a useful life, and not merely to limp along, aged and decrepit, but fit, vigorous, and virile.

Agedness can be advanced and retarded as we understand the means and causes. Ignorance is man's main crime against himself.

This book is dedicated to the man (and woman) who would live usefully and happily beyond the customary expectation.

The basis of the philosophy is, as Shakespeare said, that the fault lies not in our stars, but in ourselves. The solution to our problems is in our own knowledge and awareness.

Luck is a poor substitute for knowledge: for work. A fatalistic attitude is foolish. We can control our destiny, and many men realise that commercially.

Why not, then, our longevity, fitness and well-being? Nature has no favourites. It is true some are born stronger: sensible people take few risks. It pays to be intelligent: to avoid the pitfalls since, 'death can be so permanent'!

Chapter One

What man is: how long on Earth: the time scale: how he lived for countless centuries: caves: wild animals and stress: exercise: food.

The Scientists are reasonably agreed that man, in the form of homo sapiens, has existed upon the Earth for 1,750,000 years, or, in round figures, two million years.

During almost the whole of this time, as I will show later, man lived as a primitive animal, and much of the time without the aid of fire to cook his food, warm his body, and without tools that enabled him to build shelters, or clothe himself other than perhaps skins.

The last remnants exist in only one Continent, and that is – Australia. Here in the Great Sandy Desert, in N.W. Australia, the Aboriginal still hunts with spears, clubs and the curved boomerang, is completely unclothed, and survives without any housing other than a brush wind-break. However, he has fire, which he generates by rubbing two pieces of wood together until one smoulders, and when blown upon, ignites tinder such as the shredded bark of a tree.

He survives with none of the ailments, and despite his retreat into the aridity of the desert, and with insufficient natural subsistence, other than which is garnered under extremely arduous conditions, I repeat, he survives without any of the ailments accepted as normal for civilized man, from measles and mumps and decayed teeth, to faulty circulation or hearts, or any of the other diseases known to mankind. He dies, when not from a spear thrust, then from sheer old-age.

The Aborigine's diet is mostly flesh foods. He has to run down most of his food in the form of the Kangaroos and Wallaby. The children rouse out lizards from tufts of grass, and search for eggs: the women gather grass seeds and roots. The main element in the diet is protein, yet despite this good health is maintained and the aborigine, maybe because of the arduous nature of his life, has a good expectancy of life, even if it be but little more than the three score years and ten. I assume, on a diet largely of flesh, he suffers the relative shortness of the life-span as do most flesh-eating creatures, the carnivora having a much shorter life-span than the vegetarians of the animal kingdom, the relation in favour of the non-flesh eaters, being from double to as much as twenty times, in the case of some animals over others.

It may be of interest to record, verbatim, an account of the stamina and capacity of a young aboriginal boy, and as recorded by one of my most informed athletes. This athlete, Peter Weir, who has done much research and experimentation in proof of my ideas as to athletics, and human perambulation in particular, made several trips to the Great Sandy Desert by plane, to observe the aborigine in their natural environment. That he was able to verify the correctness as to my pronouncements on posture, walking and running, contributes something in this connection, viz.: fitness and survival other than this short statement.

So his account of the activities of a young aborigine has a direct bearing upon the case of the young civilized human being, especially as found in our cities, and in view of the fact that, in the U.S.A. and now, in Australia, almost 50 per cent of the call-ups for Military Service fail to reach the required physical and mental standards, even for National Service!

CHAPTER ONE

My athlete wrote to me under date of March 1, 1965, and I quote verbatim, from his letter (writing of modern youth):, ... but so many have lost the basic instinct ... through soft, civilized living. If only some of the younger ones could see the struggle for survival of the young aborigine generation in the Great Sandy Desert – these natural instincts would come flooding through, consciously and unconsciously through necessity – the survival of the fittest: the challenge of Nature. But they know nothing of these things ... where a young boy, to prove to himself and his tribe, hiked (and I mean hiked – running, trotting, always moving) – 80 miles, or thereabouts, chasing a young kangaroo; he lost (as far as we could tell on enquiry – it took over half an hour of persistent persuasion on my, and a local Native's part to get the information out of him and then reluctantly) his spear after 30 miles when he attempted to down it from close range; after 80 miles he ran it into the ground, what price the survival instinct? End of quote.

The interesting part of this account, to me, is how a city-bred youth, or even any European lad, would fare if he was placed in a similar position, as to survival.

It might be said that, being civilized, no such lad would be expected either to need such an instinct for survival, nor would he need to be able to survive by travelling 80 miles, apparently without food, water or rest. Yet I will submit that the exigencies of modern life demand, if not the ability to travel over desert country to the order of 80 miles, at least, a similar amount of the survival instinct, and it is because this instinct has been so lessened, in some cases, almost to the point of non-existence, that civilized man, and his well-being, is in such a parlous condition.

This, then, is the basic problem. To realise that civilised man has so departed from the primitive, and the way his ancestors lived for countless centuries, that the price he is paying for this departure is the price of incipient disease, unfitness, and basically, the lack of sufficient instinct to keep himself alive.

CHAPTER ONE

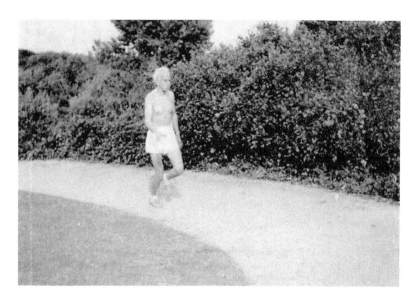

Another part of a stride in running. Note the absence of tension, the bent right knee, and the low carriage of the arms.

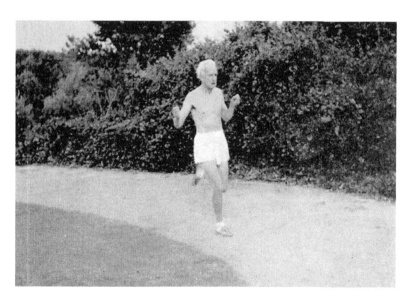

At another part of a stride. In this case the arms have come up high as the lungs are fully filled with air, something rarely seen even with world-class runners.

CHAPTER ONE

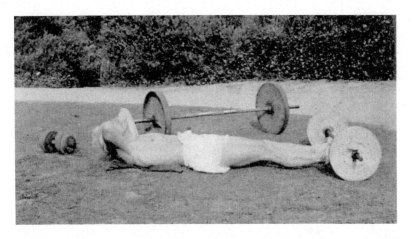

The Sit-up Exercise. At the commencement of this exercise the hands are placed behind the head, and are thus able to help force the body into the sitting position. This pressure puts tension upon the neck muscles and they benefit isometrically. Note that the feet are held down by being placed under the bar of the barbell. There is no point in attempting this exercise without the feet being held down. With the feet under a bar or a strap isometric tension is placed on the leg muscles.

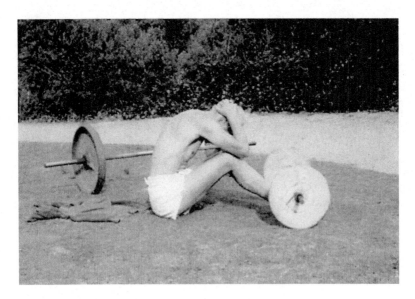

The Finish position of the Sit-up. Note that the legs have bent naturally and the head is being forced down between the raised knees. This means that the whole bodily musculature is receiving benefit from the exercise.

CHAPTER ONE

To support this argument, it is interesting to make certain comparisons. Let us, then, assume a time scale equal in distance to four feet. In doing this we accept the figures of the scientists as to man's existence on Earth.

Recorded history, that is written accounts, go back no further than 5,000 years, and 5,000 years can be considered the time when civilization, as we now know it, could be said to have commenced. But even then all Europe was still barbarian, and perhaps only half of that time ago, the inhabitants of the British Isles, for instance, were dressed in skins, and without learning other than the simple processes of the instinctive matters of procreation, killing and eating. Yet on the time scale of four feet, the last 5,000 years represents only one-eighth of an inch. The last 2,500 years a mere sixteenth of an inch, and, when we consider the last 100 years, the period only, of the modern City with its automobiles, factorised foods, and all the other amenities that have arisen, even since the turn of the century, we find that this period of intense civilization, of an order never before experienced, represents merely .0025 of an inch on our four feet time scale.

To show this point in another illustration may be justified, perhaps, because it is the fundamental reason for the state of health that modern man finds himself in, his early demise, and almost universal unfitness, at least after he attains 40 years of age.

We shall, then, take another time scale, this time we shall assume a clock, the big hand of which travels once round the face, that is, for one hour or 60 minutes. On this time scale we find that one second represents 500 years, and the last 100 years of modern civilization only one-fifth of a second, an almost negligible amount of time for the tremendous adjustments that have been necessary with our modern way of life.

When it is considered that one second ago on our time scale, there were not only no automobiles, but no railway or other mechanical transport: few roads, and humans were either

CHAPTER ONE

jolted in coaches, on horseback, or walked: that there were no factories: no gas or electricity, nothing in the way of factorised foods, no artificial manures, no refined sugars or starches, no nicotine, and little alcohol for the peasants, it begins to be realised the extraordinary changes that have occurred in man's recent environment.

It becomes even more impressive when we realise that on the four feet time scale, three feet eleven and seven-eighths inches represents primitive, uncivilized man. Or, on our clock time scale the whole hour less only a few seconds is also equal to the time our primitive ancestors roamed the earth completely uncivilized.

It can be rightly asked, what is the significance of these time scales, or are they significant at all? If this is asked as an objection, or merely out of curiosity, the answer is still most significant. Actually, the realisation of what is implied by the answer is an imperative. That is, if it is not correctly interpreted, and recognised, the resulting lack of knowledge may easily be a cause of man's eventual dissolution on Earth.

The answer, then, can be summed up, as follows: 'When the environment of an organism is markedly changed, even when the change, given time, could prove to be advantageous, any such change will tend to destroy that organism.'

It is interesting to note what Robert Louis Stevenson, himself an observer, is reported to have said about the impact of European civilization upon the Polynesian people of the Pacific and I will quote from the text-book, *Aboriginal Australians*, by Tinsdale and Lindsay. Stevenson said, ' ... Where there have been fewest changes, important or unimportant, good or bad, the race survives. Where there have been most changes, there it perishes.'

Consider then, the remarkable changes in the environmental factors of man in the last 100 years, both as to his living habits, heating, work exercise – or absence of it, abundant food, and the nature of that food. For the moment we will ignore the universal, or almost universal development of the use of nicotine, alcohol, and drugs, all of which are increasingly becoming causes of man's demise, earlier than it need be.

So, only a few seconds ago on our time scale, actually, only 150 generations, or thereabouts, man lived as a primitive in caves, walled enclosures, constantly defending himself against wild animals, in an almost constant state of fear and alarms, in a word, under constant stress due to attacks, shortage of food, the elements, and positively, without the security, regularity of aliment provision, and medication that he now enjoys. Could it be that it is these recent factors – his very security: his regular intake of food that is always there, and the absence of the natural stresses, that these are the factors bringing about his unfitness, and contributing to his diseases!

Summary of Chapter One

Man has been, in some form, on the Earth upwards of two million years. Practically the whole of this time he was uncivilized: firstly a primitive, later a barbarian.

Civilization, as we know it, is only a tick of the time scale clock, the hand of which traverses the face of the clock once. The Australian Aborigine as the last of the primitives: his regime and capacities.

The last 100 years, that of the modern industrial era, represents merely .0025 of an inch on a time scale of four feet: that the period man was a primitive living, and surviving, without any of the 'aids', of medication, or education, represents three feet eleven and seven-eighth inches of our four feet time scale.

It is axiomatic: no organism (man or any other creature, vegetation), nothing: can have its environment markedly altered and expect to survive.

CHAPTER ONE

It is this marked alteration in man's living habits – food, exercise, sedentary work, that are the factors that have reduced his capacity to live healthily and survive reasonably.

Could it be that his very security: his freedom from want: ample and daily food, and the substitution of natural stresses by the artificial stresses associated with business and ambition, his urban life, even the air he breathes, that these are the contributing factors to his ill-health, and the customary physical decline after middle-age, and often, before!

Chapter Two

Statistics: longevity: recent high averages of life expectancy due to: expectancy in animals as against man.

There is no intention to make this a chapter of statistical evidence, figures, or in any way to either influence the reader, other than to put before him a few observations, perhaps, not usually considered. It is true that the life expectancy of a baby born today is much higher than the life expectancy of a child born a century ago.

But the matter of this life expectancy is not as simple as it would appear. Let us, then, examine the conditions not a century ago, but 60 years ago, that is, in the life-time of many living now.

The facts are, if one was fortunate to survive the many infant causes of premature death, and escaped other causes in childhood and early manhood, those who survived had a better than average chance of not only reaching 70 years, but into the eighties, and some, and not just a few either, into the nineties.

Today, the expectancy of the city born and reared male, especially in the executive class, is considerably less, and probably as less as 25 per cent. This means where, had he been born a century or two ago, and survived the diseases and misadventures of childhood, he could reasonably have expected to live into the eighties. Today he cannot expect to live into the seventies, and many, not into the sixties.

CHAPTER TWO

The reason for the distortion of the statistical evidence is due, almost entirely, to the remarkable advances, in my part of the world, (Australia) by the methods of Dr Truby King, a New Zealander, and which, when adopted, almost eliminated the infant deaths in Australia and New Zealand.

These techniques, together with the immense success achieved in the practice of midwifery, means few babies are lost, the proportion being only one or two per 1,000, whereas it once was as much as 10 per cent of all the children born. Even today, the incidence of child deaths can be as high as 50 per cent in certain places and in countries such as India.

Before we move on to this aspect, I will quote my personal experience with the Commonwealth of Australia's Public Service Superannuation Fund, and of which, at one time, I was a contributor. The contributors to this fund are a considerable proportion of the male adult population of Australia, and all the members have successfully passed medical examinations upon entry into the Service. In this regard they can be considered, health and longevity expectation-wise, a select proportion of the community.

Working on the actuarial figures supplied, the Administration of the Fund expected and allowed for, expectancies of life that they were surprised to find, were not realised. Instead of almost the whole of the employees in the many Government Departments living to the retiring age, and then enjoying their Superannuation pensions for upwards of ten years, and more, after the Fund had been administered for some 25 years, it was discovered that of those who did reach the retiring ages (either 60 or 65 years according to predetermination upon entering the Service) the average period that the male contributors lived to receive their pensions, and enjoy their retirement, was two years. The women in the Service enjoyed theirs a few years longer. But since the women in the Service who remained until retiring ages were an infinitesimal number of the whole number of contributors, their influence on the figures can be ignored.

After another 25 years, I have been informed that the average has moved from two years to three years. This means that the average Civil Servant, selected, in the beginning, with good health and good longevity expectancy, does not reach the 'allotted span'.

Moreover, the wastage by sickness causing early retirement, and those who die before reaching retiring age, a not inconsiderable number, be it noted, are not taken into account in computing the average expectancy for a happy, and useful retirement.

When we consider, with this figure of an average of three years only, the influence on the average of those odd few who do live into the eighties, it will be seen that many must die before even reaching the average retirement expectancy of three years. It will be noted here that averages are rather dubious figures to work from. Like the average man in the street: the average wealth of the citizens. It may be that the average income is considered £500 per annum in wages.

But when we consider the influence of the very rich, and that not inconsiderable body of earners and investors who have incomes above £2,000, and some above £10,000 per annum, it will be seen that the average citizen, and that means the many, will have an average income far below the £500 per annum that is so smugly believed he has the good fortune to enjoy.

One more illustration to debunk the value of the 'average' and how it can confuse those who may accept statistics as the literal 'truth'. This example is personal, since it deals with my own family.

I was one of nine children. All my brothers and sisters were born in the last century as I was myself. Due to the unhygienic conditions then operating in Melbourne – no sewerage, impure water, foodstuffs infested by flies, contaminated milk, and the like, the deathrate of babies was high. In my family three of the babies died before reaching one year. However, the rest of us, surviving these childhood hazards, although I nearly made the fourth, we have survived in two cases to 80 years odd, and in two other cases into the seventies. My sister, younger than I by four years still survives.

We will assume, then, for our purposes, that the average age of longevity achieved, and a high one too, relatively, is 75 years, for my family.

Now, 75 years by six children who survived equals a total of 450 years. But nine children were born and when we divide 450 by nine, we find that the average longevity of the children born to my father and mother is – 50 years. Now: today, nine children can be born into a family, and the chances are, because of the remarkable techniques of child preservation, that all the children survive. If they average a life span of 60 years, they show an average improvement of life expectancy, at birth, over my family, of ten years. Yet none of this family, perhaps, even reached 70 years!

We will carry the matter a step further. Assume that one of our modern family did die by illness, or accident, leaving eight survivors. We then have these figures: 8 x 60 = 480 years, or an average for the nine born of 53 years, again 'proving' statistically that this fictitious family lived longer than my family lived.

This, then, is the 'catch'. Surviving adults, and that means almost all the children born, are NOT living nearly as long, nor in as good general health, for that matter, as did our ancestors who survived the incidence of child deaths and wastage.

In other words, the average today, could be, for many segments of society, especially the executive class, as low as 60 years, both in actuality and expectancy.

Since even actual survival is not the whole criterion of living, and living happily and successfully, we need to take into our consideration those who, after 45 years, or before, find they are afflicted with the ills that go hand in hand with over-weight, those who have 'hearts' and higher than normal blood-pressure, and those who are victims of the rheumatoid diseases in their many

CHAPTER TWO

forms, as well as those who have lost sexual potency and in other ways, limp through their last years, when they should, and could, be in their prime.

That this unfitness is the expectation of the many, unfortunately, is true. But there is hope: it need no longer be so. No matter how much ground has been lost, most of the ill-health can be mended, much of the unfitness turned to a healthy fitness and zestful living.

Man can be a fit, virile, potent 'animal' if he would but acquaint himself of the 'facts' of life, and the factors governing, survival.

Man, too, belongs to the 'animal' kingdom. Actually, biologically, he is more closely related to the higher apes, than these apes are to their 'brothers' of the monkey tribe. Whether we originated from a common stock is beside the point. What IS true, man has survived over a known period of some two million years evolving from animal-like ancestors with prognathous jaws and limited and receding brain areas; ancestors with longer, stronger, more hairy arms, and shorter legs than what we have evolved, and ancestors who lived solely upon foods as found in nature, exposed to the elements and with no drugs or medication since he did not require any!

Compared to other animals who have accompanied him over the span of centuries and aeons of time, he is short-lived. His closest companion, the dog, achieves sexual potency at under one year and can be considered mature at two years. The dog lives, under good conditions, for about 15 years. This gives a ratio of 15 to 1 on the sexual level, and 7 to 1 on the maturity level.

His other time immemorial companion, the horse, can be considered to achieve sexual potency under two years and physical maturity by four years. Our equine friend has an expectancy of life, when not worked to death, of – around 28 years. This again gives us the figures of, roughly, 15:1, and 7:1. Throughout the animal kingdom it is much the same. Let us examine man, modern man, in the same relationship. He achieves sexual potency around his fifteenth year, and physical maturity, not before his twenty-fifth year, when the cartilage that joins his ribs to his sternum hardens and the size of his chest-box is then fixed for the rest of his life (other than the fat or muscle he may 'plaster' upon it!).

How, then, does man's longevity factor compare with the animals and which, despite domestication, live far more naturally and instinctively than does man, their master.

We have seen that animals have, roughly, a life expectancy, bar accidents, of 15:1 from sexual potency, and 7:1 above adult maturity. Man, when he lives to 75 years has, instead of 15:1, and 7:1, as his figures, 5:1, and 3:1.

However, that is not any longer the expectancy of many. The figure is more likely to be 60 years, when his relative figures become 4:1, and 2:1, respectively.

Even to achieve 105 years, his figures are raised to only 7:1, and 4 and 1/5: 1, as against the animals we presume to feel superior to!

For man to achieve a longevity comparable to the animals he will need to double his present most optimistic expectancy, viz. 100 years, and live to something over 175 years, perhaps a double century! (shades of Hobbs, Hammond and Bradman).

Yet there are some who consider this, if not as normal, yet as possible. Perhaps a brief study of the physiology of man, his make-up, and requirements will help the many, if not to an overoptimistic 200 years, at least to what should be considered a possible 100, with the last 70 or 80 of them, mature, fit: vigorous: virile, and free from disease and premature agedness.

Summary of Chapter Two

The expectancy as to longevity today is because the wastage by infantile deaths of previous centuries has been arrested. Because of this the average longevity has been increased statistically, whilst actually, those who attain manhood, that is – survive childhood diseases, do not live as long as those who attained manhood a century ago.

In the Commonwealth of Australia Public Service Departments it was found that the average period of retirement on his Superannuation Pension was only two years. Today it is little better, if at all, than three years. For the many, then, this falls short of the three score years and ten! The average longevity of the successful executive probably not as high as 60 years. Too many, by 45 years of age, are afflicted with inefficient hearts, higher than normal blood pressures, rheumatoid diseases, loss of sexual potency and which is a factor in senility, in a word, masculine parodies of what man could, and should, be.

Man has survived over aeons of time on the simple foods as found in Nature. Yet, today, his expectation is far less than that of any other comparable animal.

In animals the relation of age to attaining sexual potency can be considered as 15:1; for man it is seldom higher than 5:1. If he dies at 60 it is merely 4:1.

Even to achieve 105 years man's relative figure is only raised to 7:1. Man has to survive for upwards of 200 years to equate the survival to procreative ability that the animals enjoy.

Chapter Three

The physiology of Man: the heart, lungs, liver and kidneys.

The four main organs without which, or when they cease to function, man ceases to survive are: the Heart; the Lungs; the Liver, and the Kidneys. All other organs are dependent upon the proper functioning of these key organs.

A man can get along in some fashion without his stomach, much of his intestines, his gall-bladder, his urinary bladder, most of his glands, but without the reasonable functioning and co-operation of the 'Big Four' he is – *non est*: finished: gone to his forefathers!

Only one of the Big Four is an organ that is directly affected by conditions external to it, and that is the lungs. The other three are more indirectly affected since they are dependent upon what is passed to them by each other, and what enters the stomach, and what is ingested by the intestinal tract.

In the case of the lungs they are subjected to good treatment or ill-treatment just as we find ourselves environmentally, or what we may inhale deliberately in the case of smoking tobacco.

Subjected to contaminated air, an atmosphere impregnated with poisons, dust, smog or other clogging and irritating atmosphere components, the lungs must suffer.

In themselves the lungs are very interesting organs and, like the heart, cannot cease to function for longer than a minute or two, without risk of death.

Made up of sponge-like material, and I have the authority for 'Medicus' on this – 'Medicus' in his excellent and easily readable book, *Know Your Body* – in a day's output the lungs, with their sponge-like substance, handle, wash and reoxygenate the 25 million red corpuscles we all should have, and which, in 24 hours means 25,000,000,000,000,000 separate washings and re-oxygenatings. Quite a fair total by anyone's calculations!

Incidentally, the lungs of the females of our species are usually much smaller than the lungs of the male, and this is the main reason for their relative poor athletic performances.

Another interesting fact, according to 'Medicus', is that our lungs are made up of some 800 million air-cells or alveoli, and the lungs, if flattened out, and the alveoli laid side by side, the lungs would cover an area of a square each side of which would measure 100 yards.

As organs the apex of each lung extends into the neck area and above the collarbone, whilst the base, or bottom rests upon the diaphragm, that little-used membrane and which plays the most important part in breathing, a fact which is so little understood by civilized man and, curiously enough, with the technique of running considered normal and natural – hardly used at all by most athletes!

How curious then that the needs of, and the treatment of, such an important organ as the lungs, is so neglected when not utterly abused.

It is assumed, if most people think about it at all, that these tiny cells have the means of rejecting all the poisons, irritants, dust, smog and smoke, that they are submitted to. It is not so much that they do clog up, that they do develop tuberculosis, cancers, pneumonia and pleurisy, but that they last out an ordinary life-time without being completely filled with dust, tars and the like, and thereby rendered completely useless.

CHAPTER THREE

In childhood the lungs are new, fresh, clean and rose-pink in colour. As man ages his lungs become dull, grey, mottled, and in the case of coal-miners – black.

Yet those who, like the Eskimo, live in a dust free atmosphere, they retain the pink colour throughout life.

Obviously, what we breathe is as important as what we eat and drink, and the movement of the diaphragm exercised, and not only that we breathe deeply and fully, but that the organs in the abdominal cavity below the diaphragm are also moved and kept in good tone. This latter is not usually realised. Possibly the muscular development of the abdominals, and the diaphragm, and the movement of these parts are the most important of the exercises a man can engage in, and the most neglected.

The situation is even worse when we consider that it is this oxygenated blood that is the fuel for the heart. So we will deal with the heart, and, because of its small size, and the tremendous job it has to do, try and realise the importance of the quality and purity of the fuel that is fed into it, and upon which it works.

Although the stomach is probably the most abused organ of the whole body, it is the heart that suffers the damage since its fuel is made up of what is placed in the stomach and the oxygenated blood that passes through the lungs.

The heart is a muscular pump. Nothing more or less. But it is the most powerful and efficient pump ever devised by man, Nature or the Creator. Roughly the size, only, of the closed fist, it contains in itself four chambers and four valves. Basically it functions in the same manner as most mechanical pumps. But where it differs from all other pumps is in its efficiency and long life.

Let us examine, firstly, what it actually is, and then, the work it does.

The heart muscle is a specially developed striated muscle, different in its nature to any other muscle in the human body. It would need to be when we examine the work it is called upon to do.

CHAPTER THREE

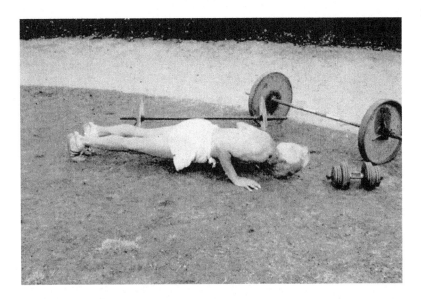

The Press-up. Another exercise that does not require apparatus. The main benefit received is the strengthening of the arms, although the whole body musculature receives benefit isometrically.

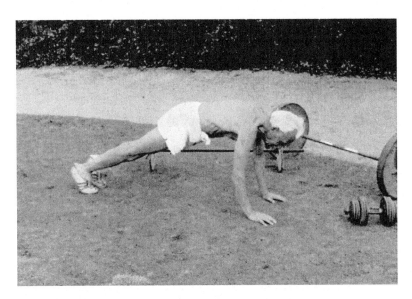

The finish of the Press-up. Note the good curvature of the body and legs, and the eyes looking down at the hands.

CHAPTER THREE

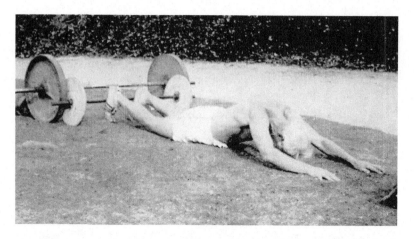

The Prone-Press. A much more difficult exercise than the Press-up. In the starting position, from laying prone on the ground, the shoulders and elbows are lifted clear and the rest of the trunk and legs follow the upward movement. This exercise is very hard to accomplish unless the feet press against a rigid object, in this case the barbell, and the hands are able to press deeply into the grass, otherwise it is best for someone to stand upon the hands to prevent them slipping forwards as the strength is exerted.

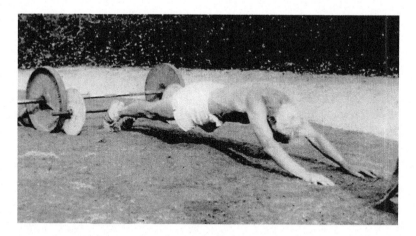

The finish of a Prone-press. The whole of the trunk and legs are clear of the ground, as must be the elbows in particular. The main stress is upon the abdominal and back muscles. The Prone-press can be considered a 'feat' perhaps more than an exercise since many otherwise strong men find they have difficulty in performing even one. Few can expect to achieve a true Prone-press at the first attempt. Fifty repetitions without a pause can be considered excellent. (The author has a best of sixty.) One hundred can be considered in the 'super' class.

CHAPTER THREE

It is interesting to note here that it carries within itself its own nervous system although it is also intimately and directly connected with the nervous system exterior to itself and which is located in the brain. Therefore, it responds to two sets of stimulations.

When we receive emotional shocks, or other causes of stimulation, the heart responds with quickened beats, poundings, slowing-ups, even missing beats! Thus has grown up the idea of the heart as the centre of the emotions. What is true is – it is intimately connected with the emotions and is a good recorder and measurer of our emotional life. But it also carries within itself the ability to know what it should do – exactly, under any set of circumstances, and without reference to the brain, and also the ability to sound warnings when it feels, or knows, it is being abused, or otherwise seriously ill-treated. Until it reaches these limits it is long-suffering and, mostly, suffers in silence.

In considering what this pump has to do we can begin to realise how important its job is, and how important it is to treat it with intelligence, care and respect.

For an organ the size it is – what it shifts in terms of weight and quantity is amazing. Its beating, or pulse rate, is usually in the order of 70 or 72 beats per minute. Each beat opens and closes all the valves and receives and delivers about 3 oz. of blood. This does not sound very much, perhaps, but it adds up to two gallons received and delivered in one minute or upwards of 100 gallons in an hour.

But that is not all. It never really stops, at least, for long, so that in twenty-four hours, whilst we forget it, ignore it or abuse it, it has pumped for us some two thousand gallons.

In a year, whilst we eat, drink, smoke and neglect to exercise it, it will be expected to handle no less than the astronomical figure of 730,000 gallons, or, if you haven't made it impossible for it to continue working for you, over your life-time of a mere 70 years – 50 million gallons of viscous fluid. Bring out your huge tankers and petrol storages. And all done with a muscular pump hardly bigger than a large orange. In an hour that pump of yours will have functioned 4,200 times. In a day 100,800 times. In a year 36,792,600 times. In your 70 years – assuming you reach that age – 2,575,482,000 operations.

For those interested in speculative calculations, as distinct from the actual facts as to an organs operation, it is calculated that the muscular energy exerted by the heart is such that it is equivalent to a prime mover raising one ton – 50 feet, over a period of 24 hours. In a year that is equivalent to lifting the ton to a height of over three miles. In 70 years, lifting the ton to a height of over 200 miles.

Another calculation suggests that the energy exerted in a life-time of 70 years would be sufficient to lift 37 tons to the top of Mount Everest. Estimations based in a calculation stated by 'Medicus' in *Know Your Body*.

But assume you have cared for this pump of yours, fed into it good fuel in the form of pure blood free of toxins, nerve and muscle drugs, and reasonably exercised it so that being strong, it can do its job pumping at the rate of 60 beats per minute, we find that over a life-time of 70 years there is a saving of 367 million pulsations as against the heart that is working at the 70 rate.

Now: that is a fair saving and we all know that when an engine, or pump, is able to work with fewer beats or revolutions, other things being equal, the machine with the fewer 'revs' lasts the longest.

But what do we find?

Due to neglect, the poisons in the fuel supply, most hearts from quite an early age have to belt it out, at a higher rate than 70, some at a rate as high as 80 beats per minute.

Assuming you are one of those whose average rate is as high as 80 pulses per minute, I am ahead of you, roughly with a margin of, around, 3,000 million beats (2,943,360,000), since my normal pulse rate is 60 per minute, and when resting has been measured by Prof. Cotton, one-time Dean of the Physiology Department of the Sydney University, when I was really fit, as low as 38 beats per minute. I was over 50 years of age, and competing in Marathons.

CHAPTER THREE

On these figures alone, since 'revs' are the basis of calculation for the life of most machines, I can expect my heart to function for me another ten years as compared with a 70 beats per minute character, and 20 years as compared with the 80 beats per minute speedster.

As I have passed into the 'Seventies' in years, with a pulse rate in the low sixties, and when really resting, below 60, in terms of heart estimations, at least, I can look forward to another 20 or SO years, other factors being equal.

But that is not the whole story. Other organs can peter out, or we, ourselves, can become fed-up with the tiresomeness of living, the futility of it all, and the rapaciousness of the tax-gatherer. Indeed, instead of being treated more and more kindly as we age, we seem to find that the ever-rising costs leave us very badly handicapped if, and when, our incomes – if any, are 'fixed', as they mostly are with the aged, and certainly are with the indigent aged! But that is by the way.

The lesson to be learned is – by and large, we are as good as our hearts and the pipes that the heart has to pump the blood through. Fortunately the routines and mechanism for maintaining the efficiency of both the pump and the pipes are now well-known. There is not, really, the slightest need for despair.

The two subsidiary organs that our life depends upon, as does the heart itself, are the liver and kidneys. Like the heart, we have only one liver. If that is mutilated, or functionally breaks down, it is the end – for it, and for us.

As well as being a vital organ it is also the largest, and I am informed it weighs about 3 ½ lb. and such is its role and importance with the blood stream, it contains, at anyone time, about one-fourth of the total amount of blood in the whole circulation.

It is, therefore, similar to a blood-soaked sponge. It deals with the material absorbed from the intestines, and is actually, just one big chemical factory. Amongst its manifold jobs, it maintains the temperature of the body, at least is a big factor in this, since it is

CHAPTER THREE

the 'boiler', the heat-producer, as it is the energy, in the form of glycogen – producer and storer.

The liver secretes, perhaps as much as two pints of bile daily. This bile is an essential, with other ferments, in the digestion of fats, and it would appear that the more fat that is ingested, the greater the amount of bile secreted.

Sugar in the form of glycogen is produced by the liver and this is the working fuel of all the muscles. But that is not enough: the liver is expected to deal with poisons that come to it in the ingested foodstuffs that find their way through our mouth via the stomach to the intestines. If these poisons are in excess the liver is really overworked, especially if it is hampered by being in an unfit condition.

Another important job of the liver is to help purify the blood, make, or help make insulin, without which you are a diabetic.

This, then, is the Liver. Unlike the stomach that can pass out of itself all the rubbish and poisons that are dropped into it, the liver has to deal with them, has no escape from its tasks and is, mostly, grossly overworked as it is most unkindly treated.

No wonder the list of diseases associated with it, and which it manfully tries to cope as it performs its functions, include Jaundice, Dropsy, Gall-stones, Cysts, Abscesses, Inflammations, Malaria, Dysentery, as well as Enlargement and Fatty degeneration. And I have left to last to mention that bane of all the good-time boys – 'Cirrhosis of the Liver'.

Cirrhosis, due mainly to the over-indulgence in alcoholic beverages, especially spirits, once changing the condition of the liver, is quite incurable. All that can be done is arrest the condition by arresting the cause, the actual tissue of the liver is replaced by a fibrous tissue and which cannot function as liver.

Obviously with too much fibrous tissue, that is, the change exceeding the needs of the body through the function of the liver, the victim must eventually die. The inability to function has exceeded the demand made upon the organ.

Now to come to the kidneys. All animals would appear to have two. They act as filters: if anything happens to one, the other can take over the entire job. So important: so sudden death is it if the kidneys cease to do the filtering for just one day that, Nature in Her Wisdom, provided two. With one, the risk would have been too great.

An excess of nitrogenous foods, that is, the proteins, flesh of all kinds, throws much work on the kidneys. They handle the urea that is got rid of by the liver. If this is not discharged into the bladder by the kidneys, Uraemia occurs I (urea in the blood) – soon a coma and death.

The kidneys, like the heart, seem to have their own nervous system or intelligence. Remarkable in their function: their ability to accept and reject the passage through them of the various substances, even the urea being sometimes retained and returned to the liver to be converted into protein.

We can be kind to our kidneys, or overwork them. It is known that an excess of nitrogenous foods (flesh foods) is rejected by the body, the sorting out, and rejection by the organism, being the job of the kidneys. It is also true that, in the absence of sufficient carbohydrates, the protein foods, by a very complicated chemical chain process, can be converted into the essential carbohydrate, and thus used as energy fuel.

In its original form, the Protein of flesh foods is not an energy food, as is so commonly believed, but is the essential body building and cell replacement blocks only.

It would appear, perhaps, that some of the by-products of excessive protein intake in the form of meat, act as a slight stimulus. Otherwise, nothing could be more fallacious than the idea that the athlete or manual worker needs more meat because of his exercise than his sedentary brother needs.

The importance of these four fundamental organs, the Heart, the Lungs, the Liver and the Kidneys, and upon which good health and longevity depends, is stressed because, if the living habits – and that means the diet, exercise, etc., are such that these organs are maintained in good health, then it can be confidently assumed that all the other organs, and physical processes, will also be in good order, and health.

If this is so then all-round fitness, general good health and maximum longevity can both be expected, and will obtain. No longer, then, will these factors of health, fitness and longevity be left to chance. The practitioner of the rules as will be set out will be one who has an intelligent interest in his well-being. This does not suggest he will live as an anchorite, a faddist or a cultist. It does imply, however, that he will be cognisant as to what lengths he can go in his self-indulgences, as well as to what extent he can ignore, or neglect his body, and still retain reasonable fitness.

Life has just as much meaning as we enjoy health and fitness and retain a zest for it. With all three factors even, the earning of a livelihood can be maintained, and enjoyed, to an age not usually thought possible.

Further, it is not inconceivable for some to find that Life – for them, only really began at 70! at which age a man could be expected to know most, if not all the answers. It can be stated that the zest will be there, even at 70, and perhaps more so – if the other two factors are fully satisfied, viz.: health and fitness.

The author assumes that the reader, by now, is ready to accept these statements, and this being so, the book will proceed upon that assumption.

Summary of Chapter Three

The four main organs upon which man's survival depends are the heart, lungs, liver and kidneys.

The lungs are the only organ directly in contact with conditions external to itself. The other organs are indirectly in contact via the stomach, and the intestines.

The lungs need to have fed into them air as pure as it is possible to obtain. The air of all great cities is contaminated by irritants and destructive gases. It is even worse when further contamination is possible through inhaling smoke from the tobacco plant with its toxic poison, nicotine, and its irritants that set up lung cancer.

The lungs have not the power of rebuilding themselves. When filled with deleterious matter, they cannot rehabilitate themselves. We breathe, therefore, live, as long as the lungs remain free from clogging substances, the treacle-like substance from tobacco, dust and similar.

The lungs are in two sections, the upper and lower as related to the entrance .of the bronchial tubes. Civilized man has increasingly lost the power of using the lower lung, requiring, as it does powerful abdominals and the full use of the diaphragm. It is the residuals that accumulate in the unused lower part of the lungs where most of the trouble occurs. Even athletes mostly run only using the upper lobes, hence they become 'winded' – and run out of wind, or air, much sooner than they need, and with impaired performances.

Without ample clean air the blood cannot be fully oxygenated. It is this blood that is the fuel to the body's pump, the heart. Without good fuel it is impossible for the heart to function as it otherwise might.

The heart is a highly specialised organ. In a natural and normal way of living it should be the last organ to cease to function. With our civilization it is mostly the first to break down and cause death.

Few people realise the tremendous amount of work that the heart is called upon to perform. In twenty-four hours – a day, and every day, it pumps some two thousand gallons of blood. Yet we ignore it, ill-treat it: starve it of good fuel, and wonder why it fails us.

The normal pulse is said to be 72. But that figure is 50 arrived at on ordinary citizens, most of whom are subnormal as to fitness they should enjoy. When an adult is really fit, and maintains his fitness for the length of his life, his resting pulse rate is found to be around 62, even lower.

CHAPTER THREE

Since any mechanical device, and the heart is a mechanical pump, is as old or worn as the use, and abuse, it is submitted to, over a life-time of 70 years, the man with a healthy pulse rate of 60 beats per minute, as against the man with 70 beats per minute, finds his heart had to beat, or work, 367 million times less. That is a huge saving in 'reps or revs' and on heart-years means that man will live at least another ten years, other factors being equal, longer than the 72 beat citizen.

Since many men, for most of their life record a pulse rate nearer 80 beats per minute, the gain to the 60-beater can be 20 years, even more.

It is obvious that a powerful, exercised, fed on good blood heart, is an asset. It could be 'the' asset.

If the life lived makes for a good strong heart, it can be taken for granted the liver will be in good order. That it needs to be in good order goes without saying if we are to live long and healthily. Apart from the congestion that can be caused with poor foods, such as animal fats, it is excess of alcohol that is the No.1 enemy, and destroyer, of the liver.

When the life lived is reasonable, the heart arid liver in good condition, it can be taken for granted that the kidneys will be in good order and functioning well. It is excessive protein foods, meat in all forms, that overtaxes the kidneys.

Be reasonable in your intake as to red meats, fish and poultry, and you are little likely to have kidney trouble, much less bladder trouble.

Life is what we make it: or how we absorb it. It is the same with our bodies; our body: our organs, glands and functions, are just as good as we intelligently feed them, exercise them, and realise that they must collapse: deteriorate: and we say – 'let us down', when from ignorance, misuse, abuse, and neglect, we let them down!

Chapter Four

The brain; mind; illusions; disillusionments and frustrations.

Probably, and I am going to put the proposition, the brain is the least part of us that we can trust. That is, the thinking part of our brain.

Because we have been highly educated, or been successful in our profession, or business, we are inclined to the idea that we are not only mostly brain, but that we have a remarkably good organ in the one we have and which we proudly feel we have developed! Because of this we almost trust it as infallible.

Just how false this assumption can be is seen when, having used our brain, gained some eminence, or wealth, we find that this brain of ours has been so unkind, so inefficient, that it has permitted us to become unfit, develop a condition where a coronary has intervened, or even worse, our brain has not warned us that a cancer has started up. It tells us when to sell shares on the Stock Exchange, how to build a Sky-Scraper, a Sputnik, and a Computer, but it does not tell us the inevitable result of the effect of nicotine, alcohol, or poor food, the importance of exercise, in a word – how to live healthily, fit and to a ripe old age!

There is a reason for this sad state of affairs.

The brain weighs about 50 ounces, or a little less. Males can take some comfort in the fact that, although the female brain, on

CHAPTER FOUR

the average, is a far more efficient one than the male, it is some five ounces lighter and thus smaller. However, not all of this bulk of brain serves us on the intellectual level. Actually, only a relatively small part, the major part of the brain has little or nothing to do with our thinking, our decisions, judgment, will, or any other of the factors that make up our personality; that causes us to believe ourselves 'clever', intellectual or superior by virtue of our gifts as artists, musicians, business men or politicians.

Often, the most highly gifted, or developed brain, can prove to be a poor one when it comes to being even normally sensible, i.e., rational functioning, as a human being. Indeed, it would often appear that the over-development of the conscious part of the brain tends to override, and thus inhibit, the normal functioning of the other part of the brain.

In a word a man with a very clever brain is not necessarily the man who is clever enough to realise, or appreciate, even the simplest of things as they may relate to his health, fitness, longevity, and well-being generally.

The brain is made up of several lobes or chambers, each separate from another and what is considered the thinking part, the part responsible for our intellectual, emotional, and self-conscious life is established in the grey matter of the brain. This grey matter is only a small part. The greater part of the brain being white matter. The whole of the brain is said to be made up of nine thousand million cells, (9,000,000,000), if that helps.

Moreover, the area of the brain devoted to sensation, hearing, memory and the like, is far greater than the area considered the seat of our thinking and intellectualism.

However, there may be some consolation in the fact that clever people have cells in the thinking part of the brain that are greater in size and number than the cells found in idiots. It is also flattering to know that the lower animals, even monkeys, have none of these cells, only our Kinsman, the higher apes have any, and then, not a great many in comparison with man.

Another interesting aspect is that various parts of the brain function independently of other parts. Thus, injury to one part need not imply injury to other parts. In other words, a man can have an injury that paralyses his mobility but need not necessarily affect his conscious thinking.

It is also pertinent to remember that memory is a function of part of the brain, and the area where memory is said to reside is not part of the area where thinking and intelligence is said to function. This is true of the faculty for calculation.

It also means that, to have a memory that can absorb and repeat countless facts, or, even, to be acclaimed as a scientific or mathematical genius, does not mean that the intelligence part of the brain is one iota greater than many a very ordinary, undistinguished citizen.

This accounts for the sometimes extraordinarily foolish behaviour of people assumed to be highly gifted, intellectual, and that a wisdom and native sagacity is often found, not only in people who have not demonstrated great intellectual capacity in the sciences, but by people who may be illiterate, as we find when a native chieftain outwits a learned diplomat.

Thus it is that we find it is not erudition that keeps the medical man fit, healthy and alive (actually they often die earlier than their patients) – but the native, or inborn sagacity, call it wisdom, that guides, through the instincts, those who survive from those who do not survive.

Another factor that is relevant to our proposition is the influence exerted upon our behaviour by the conditioned, or unconditioned, response.

What we know of this important aspect we mostly owe to Pavlov.

Therefore, it is most important what habits we form, and just how intelligent our response to the various conditions imposed upon us by the civilization we find ourselves projected into.

CHAPTER FOUR

Summed up, we can take the brain for granted: neither rejecting its conscious decisions, nor accepting them. At the best the conscious mind can only absorb and use what is put into it, true or untrue. In itself the conscious mind has no power to determine what is true, and what is untrue. It is the unconscious part of the brain, the part in which the instincts are situated that can be more reasonably trusted to guide us to what is true and what is untrue. However, it is when the unconscious and instinctive part is not powerfully developed, or worse, has a low I.Q. as an inherited factor, that, when the conscious part is seized upon early in a child's life that the most extraordinary ideas, as a conditioned response, can be imposed upon the mind.

This is so obviously true in the teachings of religion, as well as philosophy, that we have countless millions of adherents, each believing his beliefs to be true, but with beliefs diametrically opposed to one anothers, and of the most extraordinary, and irrational order.

Where the instinct is well-developed, all or most of the teachings that condition the mind of the many will be instinctively rejected, although the conscious mind, especially in the case of a child, will neither know, or be able to suggest a reason for the rejection.

Actually, this is the test for inborn fundamental wisdom, and intelligence, and something which is entirely apart, or separated from conditioned intellectual learning, even when it is of the highest order.

This is the reason why we so often see the extraordinary anomaly of a mind highly intellectually cultivated, but the person believing in the most extraordinarily unscientific beliefs as those with religious adherences must believe in. When we translate this condition to the gifted surgeon, or the immensely successful business man, and many such-like greatly successful men, but who confuse us by so little understanding the simple facts of existence, or who show so little of the quality that the Greeks called 'Nous', that they die, sometimes before even 50 years of age, and almost always from normally preventable diseases, or neglect of, or abuse of, their bodies.

It is not necessarily fate, destiny or luck, that some people live whilst others die. Even in the case of many who live with a history of sickness due to the inheritance of physical bodies inferior in the beginning to those who would appear to bear a charmed life, illness-wise.

Whilst it is an advantage to inherit a good physical body, resistant to disease, and free from inherited disabilities such as the many congenital conditions, asthma, the migraine factor, or similar, it is far more important that the person inherit an inborn instinct for survival, a natural 'Nous', and an instinctive response, developed to a high degree, perhaps, by observation and experience, of innate intelligence, wisdom and commonsense.

Such an innate intelligence or instinct guides the possessor away from the customary pitfalls whether of the physical body, or those of the personality, such as, conceit: over-ambition: intellectual arrogance: relying upon wealth and/or power, and many more unreliable 'props' that are foreign to simple, primitive Nature, and to whom, in the end, we must accord our lives, as we acknowledge Her Laws and Justice. How sad: what an end to an otherwise successful life that we arrive at 50, or 60 years of age, only to realise that we have been fooled, or that we have earned and acquired wealth: fame: success, but have not fit, vigorous, virile good health.

What frustrations this must engender. We have the financial means: the desire, but not the ability to satisfy. We see the goal, but cannot gain it. We can buy, but cannot use!

Actually, no belief in hereafters: no substitutions in heavens: no satisfactions in the past: no hopes for the future, can ever equate the moment of truth in the present when we realise we have been found wanting, as a 'man': that we are mainly, not a complete fully functioning physical organism, but merely a 'brain' that stands in front of a huge amount of money, great quantities of assets, or whilst we live, the power to issue commands to others.

None of these things can ever equate the satisfaction of feeling in our self-fronting moments: in our moment of self-revelation: that we are still a complete man: our organs sound: our muscles strong: our glands functioning: and, above all, interesting to women because of our accepted and recognised capacities.

Summary of Chapter Four

Because we have been highly educated, or successful in business, or our profession, it does not mean that our brain can be trusted to warn us, direct us, or guard us, when it comes to fit, sensible, and healthy living.

Indeed, if we look at most of our contemporaries, it is obvious their brain is doing little for them in safeguarding them from coronaries and cancers.

The reason is that the intelligent, the 'thinking' part of the brain, the grey matter, is a relatively small area of the brain. Much of the other part is useless to help us consciously, or we would all be in first-class health: fit as trouts: and living happily and healthily to one hundred, at least!

'Clever' brains are not necessarily wise or highly intelligent brains. In fact, to be too clever in some fields can be a trap, since we are inclined to assume we are clever in all the varied departments of living. A genius dead at 44 betrays that illusion.

The brain does not guard us, instinctively, as to our environment since, possibly, if it did, no one would smoke, drink alcohol, eat denatured foods, or live in air-contaminated cities.

However, we can keep alive the instinctive part of our brain and learn to listen to its promptings.

It is not necessarily fate, or bad luck, that some die, whilst others live. Actually, a long and reasonably healthy life is a result of instinctive wisdom, experience, and nous, much more than most folk realise. Seldom is it due to the work of doctors and surgeons after we have broken down.

We do not have to die, otherwise rich or successful at 60, much less 50. Indeed, it is the rich and successful who have the means to make long life and fitness certain.

Substitutions, such as hereafters, even endowments and security, can never equate the feeling of fitness, and realising that we have strong muscles and functioning glands. No natural door or function need be closed to any fit man, even when 70 and 80. That much has been proved.

Chapter Five

Life as a challenge: repressing emotion and the blood pressure: stress and ulcers.

All men of spirit and intelligence accept the life they find themselves in as a challenge. Too much is made of ambition. No child is born ambitious. Most children are born competitive. The instinct to struggle for survival: a place in the society a child finds itself in, is innate in all of us, almost without exception. How we receive this challenge influences our later to-be-developed ambition.

Unfortunately, born with a good physical body and discovering within himself an above average brain, the normally ambitious man, and women, for that matter, sets out and deliberately, to equate that ambition as it is first aroused in him, and later, from time to time, since, even in the greatest of ambitions, although the mind may conceive, or imagine the ultimate possibilities, it is only by travelling step by step, day by day, that any man ever achieved his ambition, great or small.

But I said 'unfortunately', since it is to be regretted that the ambition of men almost invariably excludes a well-devised, or thought-out plan for maintaining a first-class physically fit, vigorous and virile body.

At the most, greatly ambitious, moderately ambitious, or men with little or no ambition in the accepted sense, all alike tend to ignore the demands and needs of the physical. Many, since they find a need for relaxation, or escape, use their bodies as the means, not to escape or find relaxation, as they well might in arduous physical activities and feats, but in abusing it through over-indulgence in rich and unnecessary foods, and excessive quantities of alcohol. Both can be eventually fatal, at least, as to the 'death' of any real ability, or capacity, for a life of vigour, and zestful physical enjoyments.

Mostly, by 40 years of age, such men have lost all sense of satisfaction, if they ever permitted themselves to find the time to enjoy such pleasures, as in long walks in the mountains, even walking at all, swimming and diving, or a daily regime that involves some sweating exercise, and not so much as a 'medicine', a drill, or a task to be endured, but because they still retain enough youthfulness, a sense of 'play' and zest, that they derive real pleasure from these pursuits.

It is true many indulge in some weekly golf, even squash and tennis, and an occasional swim. Some sit in boats and fish, even sail boats. Most, however, watch others exercise as spectators at football, or the horse races, and even in this latter, it is mainly the idea of combining a little pleasure with the hope of acquiring some more wealth, washed down by some aqua vitae.

None of these things, as mostly enjoyed, are the complete way to masculine fitness and virility: much more is ordinarily required.

It is even worse when, in accordance with our ambitions, and because the many, as ourselves, mostly ignore the realities and conform to the status quo, we find that, to succeed largely, we have to suppress our instinctive and natural emotions. Let us examine the picture as it mostly presents itself.

All, most anyway, ambitious and successful men, as well as many not so ambitious or successful, find themselves thrown into the company of the females of the sex, in a thousand different ways, from Secretaries and Manageresses, to the various employees down to the girl who makes their cup of tea.

CHAPTER FIVE

Business, and ambition, makes it impossible for men who come in daily contact with such females to express their feelings as they might otherwise do. So they learn, and practice emotional repression. They learn to ignore the sex as such (except, perhaps, in some odd special cases!) and in this way condition themselves to states of repression that must, and do, have an adverse effect upon their emotional life, and through it, their glands and secretions.

It is axiomatic, at least in my view, that repression of any kind has an adverse effect upon the organism both as to the personality as well as physically. Yet I am not suggesting an uninhibited animal-like attitude that looks upon every female as an object of desire. But I do suggest that, instead of repressing, blotting-out almost from consciousness, the very existence of these females, that they be frankly accepted. This acceptance, however, to be successfully accomplished without the sense of frustrated desires and, perhaps, time-consuming longings, must be sublimated. This is done simply by putting the good of the woman first; instead of the woman being viewed as a unit, or female, to be exploited, either emotionally or commercially, that she be viewed as a human being whose best interests are your best interests: her happiness your happiness: her misfortunes something that you do all in your power to minimise.

Such an attitude, in business, can produce, women being what they are, responses in devotion, loyalty and work that can be amongst the most rewarding in any successful man's career. The man's ability is itself enhanced since he himself labours not merely for his own success and gratification, but that of others.

I freely admit that many employers and executives have some such attitudes to their employees, and through their various organisations, to society in general, but these relationships are too often still too impersonal when it comes to the hour to hour, and day to day, associations. In a word the older man, fit and virile as he may be, must engender a loving, but patriarchal, attitude

CHAPTER FIVE

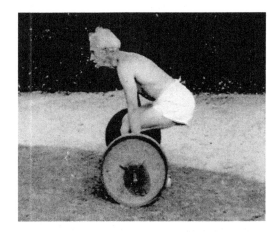

The side view shows the correct position and the angle of the body, the straightness of the back, and the gaze looking ahead. These are important details if strains and hurts are to be avoided with heavy lifting.

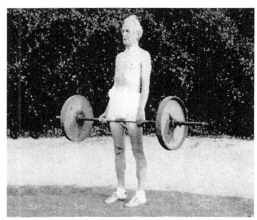

The finish of the Dead-lift. Note the stretched-up posture and the absence of strain or tension.

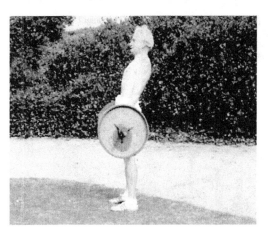

Side view of the finish of the Dead-lift. The shoulders are pulled back until the shoulder blades meet. Thus all the musculature receives some benefit from the lift. Except for the arms which are exercised isometrically, the rest of the musculature is exercised isotonically.

CHAPTER FIVE

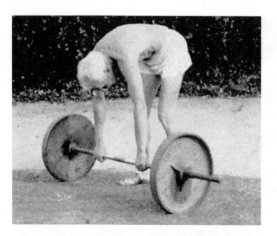

The Dead-lift. This picture demonstrates the wrong way to attempt to lift anything at all, and not only a heavy barbell. There is not one single thing right in such a position and which can be expected to cause, when the weight is heavy enough, strains, displacements, even ruptures.

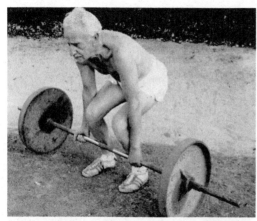

The Dead-lift performed the correct way. Note the bent knees close to the bar, the feet under the weight to be lifted, the flat back and at a 45 degree angle from the horizontal, and the grip of the hands, one hand over and one under, on the bar. The feet are placed well apart.

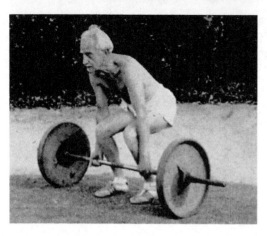

The weight about to leave the ground. The head has come up a little as the strain is fully taken. Note how the legs are inside the arms and that the position is as if sitting.

CHAPTER FIVE

to the women he is confronted with in his business associations. Otherwise stresses, conscious or unconscious, are set up in his organism and these can be reflected in his physical well-being as well as in his substituted appetites.

Another cause of emotional repression is when the man of affairs realises that, if he gives way to his reasonably emotional responses, especially the emotions of anger, impatience or dislike, that he will inhibit his prospects. That man, by learning, and practising too great a self-control, may advance his business or other worldly interests, but he will as assuredly create emotional tensions within himself and which, when translated to the physical, cause those digestive disturbances, tensions and stresses which, when they do not directly affect the action of his heart and his blood pressure, can be believed to be a factor that can result in his ulcers, even, and it is not impossible, his tumours and cancers.

Not that I suggest such ulcers and tumours, are caused directly by the tensions and stresses involved in modern civilized living, but I do suggest that these tensions may affect the functioning of the digestion itself, as well as create artificial hungers (and thirsts) and these, in the form of ignorant, or careless, eating; can be the direct cause, at least of the peptic ulcers so commonplace, but needlessly so.

Time and again I have seen men struggling to swallow their anger, even righteous anger, and pretend to a good will they far from feel. My advice is – never be one who consciously swallows his anger when he feels impelled to speak out, cost him what it will. (The actual swallowing of the Saliva takes place.) I am not suggesting that any man gives vent to his feelings like some unintelligent tyro, but if he expresses his emotional feeling, and deeply feels he is justified in his attitudes, he will mostly find, not only will he not engender ulcers or blood-pressures, but that he will become more respected; perhaps, if he wishes it, more greatly feared.

CHAPTER FIVE

Even if this does not eventuate, it is better to lose the argument, proposition, or possibilities, than risk the possibility of harming the physical organism, as continued repression well might. In any case, I have observed that what we may term the 'biggest' men, the most successful, whilst they may not give way to a show of emotion confronted with the many tiring, but often only petty, occurrences, it is not that they repress their emotion, but that they ride the petty with intelligence and ability.

But when a 'real' situation calls forth the need for plain speaking, even an emotional outburst, they are not found wanting in their expression, whether win or lose. Anyway, they invariably win!

Man has always lived under emotional tension, mostly the emotion of fear. He still has fear as his most potent cause of stress.

If we analyse life it is mostly fear that motivates us. In primitive times, man lived in constant fear, if not actual seasonal or random occasions of starvation, then fear of enemies, wild beasts, the unknown, and fear of his chiefs, medicine men, as well as fear of loss of status, and much else, just as modern man experiences in his society today. All these states are normal. They created stress, tensions and conditions similar, or more so, than today. Yet primitive man did not develop 'hearts', coronaries, high blood pressures, or any of the other disabilities that modern man suffers from. Modern man, then, must look elsewhere for these causes of his ill-health, and his, too often, sudden and premature departure from our midst. This book will unfold these causes. The preventions, even hopefully, suggest the 'cures'. Let it be so.

Summary of Chapter Five

Accept life as a challenge. Yet keep ambition within reasonable attainment. It is far more sensible to enjoy a full and happy life than to be the busiest, richest, and most successful man in your City, much less in that City's cemetery.

Being over-ambitious can destroy since it leaves the over-ambitious man little time to live: to know: to realise.

The demands and needs of the physical body cannot be ignored. A lip-service to exercise, i.e. weekly golf, or a fishing excursion, is not good enough.

The instinctive demands should be listened to: never entirely repressed out of consciousness.

Life is to be lived: not just laboured through. Repression stultifies life: Expression enjoys life. Women are 50 per cent of our environment: learn to live with them: love them: serve them. It is a policy that pays off. Exploitation of anything, especially women, never did pay. Nature is on their side: not yours.

It is bad to swallow, actually to go through the act of swallowing one's saliva, or tonsils, as it were – when angered, or otherwise aroused emotionally. Whilst it is not suggested that an adult male give way to every humour and respond to every pettiness, it is suggested that, when things are vital: important: even hazardous, it is far better, in the long run, to express your feelings than repress them.

At that Board Meeting: that Party Meeting: in Conference with your boss: if it looks as if plain speaking: repudiation: cost you what it may, in promotions: status or loss of leadership even, it will be found to payoff in the long run.

There is a 'law' involved in all this: action and reaction. Standing up for a principle: justifiable anger, especially when it is for a non-personal reason, wins the support and respect of the worthwhile even when such support and respect are not covert.

At least one will 'feel' a man: and, perhaps, live to learn one has become a 'bigger' man. We all live in, and with fear. Fear crates stress and tension. Learn to turn fear to your account: enlist it in your service: when we understand and overcome, fear, we overcome most things that tend to kill us.

Actually, it is fear, rather than ambition, or duty, that causes us to work so: to ignore so much: and which ends up in our coronaries: heart attacks: ulcers and other ills of so many 'successful' men.

Make a decision: express yourself: take your holiday. After all, it will all be the same in a hundred years. There is no true success where there is ill-health, or sub-health, or a lessening of human masculine functions.

Chapter Six

The chief destroyers: de-natured foods: nicotine, not worry: alcohol, not over-work: barbiturates (sleeping pills, sedatives – even aspirin, and the like): gambling a cause of stress

Undoubtedly, and in my considered opinion, it is the food that modern man feeds into his digestive tract that is the cause of many, if not most, of his ills. In a later chapter, the type of food he must eat will be fully discussed. For the moment, we shall then deal with the 'extras' to his food intake, and which have become a normal part, hardly to be questioned as to whether they are good or bad for him, their use being taken so much for granted. We shall examine nicotine.

Until the beginning of this century tobacco was not as universally used as now, and its consumption was almost exclusively in the form of the cigar and pipe-smoking. In this form the extract from tobacco, the powerful drug, nicotine, entered the system by absorption in the mouth, and, when swallowed with the saliva, by absorption in the stomach and/or the intestines. Cigarettes, and inhaling of the smoke to the lungs was little known.

Today, the practice of smoking cigarettes, and inhaling is, perhaps, the most general form of ill-health and poor levels of fitness, when it is not a direct cause of death.

Nicotine is readily oxidized and much of its potency escapes when submitted to heat, otherwise the quantity in only one packet of cigarette could be sufficient to cause death.

However, sufficient of the poising is contained in the smoke arising from the combustion, that the inhalation of the smoke into the lungs has sufficient stimulus to advance the heart beat from four beats to 14 beats per minute. For the person who may 20 or 30 cigarettes a day this result on the heart will be found, since it is not yet recognized by 'the profession' as one of the main causes of heart disease, notably Angina.

It is the irritants in this smoke, and not the drug itself, the tars and other products of Combustion, that are the chief causes of lung cancer. That habitual inhalation of the smoke from tobacco causes lung cancer is no longer doubted or denied. but then the tars and irritants from inhaling auto-mobile exhausts, and many other of the fumes, especially those arising from coal tar, all these cause cancer o f the lungs.

Incidentally any product from coal-tar, colouring matter, flavourings and the like, carry with them the cancer inciting irritant. These things are known, even if vested interests deny them, as they do.

Cigar and pipe-smoking, with the juices as well as the smoke taken into the mouth, are a cause of lip, mouth and throat cancers, as they cause cancers in the stomach. No less an able man than Sigmund Freud, the Father of Modern Psychiatry, died from cancer of the mouth due his habit of cigar smoking.

The late King George, it is said, was warned that he would die prematurely, if he did not give up smoking.. The list of notable people is endless.

The Nicotine is a stimulant since it markedly increases the action of the heart. But two minutes vigorous exercise would do the job better, wake us up, and without any risk at all to our health, exercise being natural.

CHAPTER SIX

The dictum is clear: adamant: and permits of no more procrastination. Quit smoking! It is true, some get away with it, or appear to, and man quote Sir Winston Churchill. One man in a thousand perhaps[1] consider those you know: fiends, business associates and who didn't reach 90! Because of its potency as a drug, it is hard, very hard, and for some men, impossible to relinquish the habit. That is the challenge. Beaten by an ounce of tobacco, or a packet of cigarettes. It is sad, but true, the moral and physical weakness of many men. Certainly it is worth the effort. Once overcome – the appetite, general health and well-being improves, as some experience, remarkably.

It is the drug, Nicotine, that inhibits good digestion. The day will come when the circulation of the poisons from tobacco in the blood stream, will be recognized much ore than it is now, as a probably cause of cancer in various parts of the body, and not just in the lungs, mouth and throat.

It is a foul-smelling habit, anyway. Fortunately, it would appear to affect fecundity so that the desire for sexual intercourse tends to abate with the regular consumption of the drug over years. Thus, nice women, sensitive to the horrible breath and general odour of the tobacco – redolent lover, repellant as this must be, are spared from a too frequent onslaught upon them.

No matter how fit you may be: how virile: how potent – assuredly you will be fitter, more virile: more potent once you conquer your addition to the drug Nicotine, as you will be if you have other addictions, and conquer them.

Addict or not, this is certain, the Nicotine addict must and does, shorten his life, and by years, especially the cigarette addict. Then, with this overcoming for most, anyway, is found that all overcomings are relatively easy. No addict to anything surely, can

---

[1] It is known that in the last decade of his life Winston Churchill suffered two strokes and was, generally, a very sick, unfit man.

CHAPTER SIX

view himself as a real, self-determining man! Nr can he achieve the respect, not only of himself, but of others.

Again, if you are addict, Quit! Despite its obvious results when a person is intoxicated, or when he has achieved cirrhosis of the liver, Alcohol unlike Nicotine, and other drugs of modern use, has been a part of civilization, even of primitive life, from time immemorial. Wine is mentioned in the Bible, and whilst there are warnings against it, its use is not actually forbidden.

Thus it is that mankind has developed some kind of tolerance, and which Nicotine has not yet had time to develop, if it ever does.

Alcohol, even in excess, does little damage to the heart. Actually, in moderation, it is useful to the heart since it slows down its action. The increased pulse rate due to the exigencies of the business world, is reduced when alcohol is taken. It is, in itself, a depressive, i.e., has a sedative action. The 'loose tongue' so often noticed after some alcoholic intake is not due to any stimulus, but is due to the sedative effect of alcohol upon certain inhibitive centres of the brain.

This, in itself, is not harmful, since it can reduce tension, and brig about a respite from the stresses that beset all workers, whether brain or physical.

The use of alcohol, like all palliatives, is reasonably justified until the user has become habitual in its use, or excessive. Excess use of alcohol is to be deplored, perhaps more because of the effect upon others, the accidents that following its train, and the domestic unhappiness.

What is not generally appreciated is what happens when nicotine and alcohol are taken into the system simultaneously. The one acts as a stimulus to the heart, the other a s a sedative just how the heart feels about it , and deals with these conflicting drugs, it does not say, but in the view of the facts, the use of both, especially at the same time, does seem a little anomalous, to say the

CHAPTER SIX

least! But then man was never really noted for his sanity.

The rise in the use of the pain-killing, and sleep inducing drugs is another cause for wonder, in view of man's declining physical well being.

Only recently has it been observed that the use, other than in very moderate does, of the common aspirin, is a cause of bleeding of the stomach. It is comforting to know that some medical authorities consider a modicum of stomach bleeding as quite okay, not serious: nothing to be alarmed at!

Frankly, and across my heart, I would not be happy to know that my stomach bled from any cause whatsoever. Anything that causes internal bleeding must be suspect.

I hold that it is evidence of a decadent society when men and women resort to the pain-killers, the acid-neutralizers, the bowel-movers, and the many other pills, powders and medications that re now so commonly used.

Undoubtedly the aim should be to live without any of these adventitious aids, since not one of them can be considered advantageous to the organism, n matter how beneficial they may be considered in righting the chronic ills modern man seems to have become heir to. The advice here is Learn to Live without them!. And in the case of alcohol, make sure your intake is within the limits of your personal tolerance, and this tolerance exists differently for each person. Therefore, no attempt is made to lay down quantities. However, this much is certain: alcohol in too 'neat' a form is definitely more harmful to the organs than the same quantity in a more diffused form. Spirits, I believe, can take a greater toll of the organism than ales and beer, and both, probably, more than wines.

However, there is no question at all, no matter in what form alcohol is imbibed, if it is in excess of the tolerance of an individual, its results are classic. No one can live with a liver than has changed its nature. In extreme cases, the brain also, can be affected, and finally the sexual potency.

CHAPTER SIX

It would seem strange to many that gambling is dealt with in the same chapter as drugs and soporifics. But that is just what gambling, in its nature is – a form of soporific.

The chronic gambler lulls his sensibilities into a kid of coma in which he trusts to his luck, chance or fate. He 'backs' his fancy and his judgment, whether it be on the Stock Exchange, the Race-course, the Gaming Table, instead of backing himself, and his ability to win-out, without the adventitious help of Lady Luck.

Whilst it is true that many gamblers may appear to succeed financially, nothing is ever gained without a price being paid, and the high tensions and stresses experience by the habitual gambler in no way aid him, to enjoying perfect health, even long life.

In perfect, or almost perfect health, there is a disregard of the idea of gaining without earning, and that is what gambling implies. It is true many see so little chance of achieving anything worthwhile, especially financially, other than through gambling, the sweepstake, or some other form, that there may be some justification for such forms of speculation. But other than such people, and for them, too, it is a confession of defeat, or inability to earn by labour, whether of the brain or body; or it is desire to gain at the expense of another. No fit, vigorous and, must I say it, sensible man, would rely upon gambling as the main means of achieving his ends, winning out in life, or demonstrating his manliness.

In this respect gambling is as much a disease, a sickness as any other form of personality, or mental illness. Psychologically, it is related to suicide.

I make a distinction where a man, because of his belief in himself, whether it be playing a game, some feat of exertion or work, is prepared to back himself., I have often done so myself, but, gambling on the turn of a card, two flies on a window pane, even to anticipating the trend of affairs on the Stock and Share Market, or the Race-course, when indulged in as a livelihood, or the main part of a livelihood, suggests that as a man, we are prepared to let others do the work, whilst we gamble upon the result of it.

I feel gambling as such, damages the personality and that, even apart from tensions and stresses, and any possible effect upon the physical organism, is to be deplored. At all costs a man should aim to be a man.

This is no morality. I view it as a factor in zest, self confidence, masculinity, in a word, being a 'full' man: a complete personality: a responsible and usefully contributing citizen.

That I feel that all these factors are tied in with a fit body is true. When the personality is thrown back upon itself: when it is realized that there is only one way to a full, health, useful, disease-free life: then I opine society, meaning mankind, will tend to act differently.

And since living zestfully, fully and healthily, rather than mean a contracting lie, makes for an expanding life – more of everything from the enjoyment of exercise, change and travel, through all the arts to the enjoyment of women, then I feel some reasonable attitude to fitness is soundly justified. After all, only the fit are fearless: and only fit lovers make love. Wealth and honours may be compensations – never substitutions.

Summary of Chapter Six

Man is the food he eats: the fluids he drinks, and the air he breathes. Let all three be poor, denatured, contaminated, and he must be less fit and healthy than he otherwise could be.

Tobacco is the prime killer today, although it will be some years before its action is fully realized by the 'profession'. Vested interests are still too powerful. But you needed be the victim: the sucker.

The Nicotine in tobacco is the drug that affects the heart. It is the tars and other irritants in the smoke that causes lung cancer. However, although no proved as yet these irritants circulating in the blood streams ay well cause tumours and cancers in other parts of the body. Certainly the juice of tobacco causes mouth, throat and stomach cancer.

Alcohol in excess, and each man's tolerance varies, and very considerably in some cases, can cause death through cirrhosis of the liver. Otherwise alcohol in excess is a social evil. In moderation, alcohol is kind to the heart, reduces the pulse rate, relieves tension, and even, perhaps, helps to make us more human, more easy to live with.

Alcohol is a sedative, a depressive. Nicotine and excitant and stimulant: how foolish to imbibe both simultaneously.

The modern drugs, pain kills: sedatives: tranquilizers and sleep inducers, on that rare occasion may be justified. The habitual use, and they all are habit forming – surely are not the things masculine men will be found to resort to.

Gambling can be a disease. When a business it is a social evil, it is an attempt to replace honest work by reliance upon chance, 'cleverness'. Gambling never produced anything. It is justifiable to 'back' oneself in what one does, but not in what someone else does, or even, what the share-market does. Avoid the stresses and tensions of reckless, or desperate, gambling.

Investment is one thing. Gambling in the pure sense, if we can call it that, is not likely to lead to fitness or health, either of the body or mind. Real men never did rely upon pure chance to achieve their ends. They planned and worked for certainties, or near certainties.

Chapter Seven

A sound basic philosophy is necessary: the need to recognise what life is: realism and religion: self reliance and saviours: wealth: privileges: investments: even pensions – can disappear: fitness can always be there.

There are two attitudes of mind, especially, that the older man must guard against. The one is – living in the past: his accomplishments of Yesteryear: fantasies as to his boyhood: his athletic or sporting successes: his high-marked examinations. To do this is to admit failure as to the present.

In his age group there are still 'championships' to be won: feats of strength even outdoing the young: capacities and demonstrations just as good as he ever enjoyed, since all things are relative.

The other is – projecting himself too much into the future: sacrificing today for a perhaps, nebulous, tomorrow. There must be balance.

Too many men have worked ceaselessly in order that they can enjoy the reward at 50, or 60, only to find that through lack of 'practice', that is, keeping alive from week to week the thing they look forward to enjoying, they have lost the capacity for that particular form of enjoyment.

It can be anything from gardening to travel: music to a too long postponed hobby: the enjoyment of the society of women – the lot.

CHAPTER SEVEN

The Bible refers to the need to keep our talents working and not burying them. Dr Toynbee, the noted historian, is reported to have said 'All-roundness was the Key'. And he quotes the various interests, 'all roundedness' in the lives of men such as Smuts, Einstein and Churchill.

Toynbee says that his conviction was that 'human affairs do not become intelligible until they are seen as a 'whole'. I feel strongly that business men, politicians, professional men, indeed, all brain workers, need to realise the importance of the full, rounded, complete life, and a life that includes all aspects, especially that of health and exercise, and the necessity to make the time to enjoy the various arts and culture, as well as time for quietness and cogitation.

This theme will be developed in a later chapter. Sufficient for the moment is that the busy man needs to recognise that it is not the intensity of his effort over, say, 20 or so years, but the results of his efforts, perhaps more reasonably applied, over 40 or 50 years that can be of the greatest productivity.

This fact is causing concern to many top ranking Executives in many countries. Brilliant men trained for years, and with an expectation of a life-time of service, being lost to the enterprise after only 15 or 20 years of the high-grade usefulness.

There is little sense in dying for a cause. It is far more sensible to 'live' for it. Dead men do no useful work. Unfit men slow down the community pace, even if the time lost is no more than the regular attendance at funerals.

An 'all-round' philosophy is required. It is not good enough to be almost completely ignorant about any aspect of our life and business. It is not sound practice to have to rely completely upon the judgment of another: the word of the expert. This is even more important when the ignorance has to do with self: what man is: how he functions – or should function.

In any case, whatever the attitude the approach to any problem, or difficulty, must be through the mind. In the matter of health and fitness, as in any other successful venture, the person must feel the need, the real and pressing need, for what he aims at, otherwise, most of his 'aims' will be found to be 'wishful thinking'.

Unless there is 'feeling', a deep inner need and desire, a real interest, there will not be sufficient enthusiasm to carry through with the project, whatever it may be. The Will only functions as an expression of feeling. Of itself, it is useless, since we cannot will to will.

Where there is an emotional content the will will be aroused, and remain dominant, just as long as we are still emotionally motivated. In this regard, the intellect per se, whilst accepting a proposition, does not necessarily provide the will to carry out the demands of that proposition, no matter of what order, or urgency.

A real fright arising from a slight heart attack, has put more men on the track of sensible living than all the intellectual arguments ever presented.

But the thoughtful man does not require a heart seizure, or an ulcer, or some other frightening or incapacitating experience to arouse him sufficiently emotionally to act. He can observe others, and by accepting the deep thought aroused, if he will accept it, instead of, as so many do, rationalise the happening and which can only be of the order of superficial thinking, he will say: 'If this is not to happen to me, or if I am not to risk this happening to me, I will have to do something about it'.

This is the attitude that I, the author, wish so sincerely, to arouse in the mind of my readers. The idea, not to wait for the hour of denouement: the moment of truth: the pronouncement: or the good or bad prognosis: but, by feeling: emotion: to arouse the intellect so that it, and the will, come into play.

Life can, and should be, better 'further on'. How pitiable, really, to be one who continually laments the present: has little or no hope for the future: and lives in successes, the pleasures and joys, only of the past.

CHAPTER SEVEN

It is no wonder that the philosophies that project hereafters, heavens and houris, find credence. After all, they can only be compensations for things missed in this life. The Negro spirituals came into existence out of the misery of the present, and the only hope that the slave could envisage, 'The Glory Road'. 'All God's Children got shoes', and 'I'm going to walk all over God's heaven', 'I got a Robe', and many others testify that these hopes and longings, and beliefs, grow out of nothing more scientific than hopelessness and misery.

Therefore, it should be clear that the education of the mind, the philosophy of living fully, must first be tackled, since both are neglected subjects in the life and education in the usual experience, and whether he remain in the lower bracket of financial affluence, and whether he finds his outlets in his work, spectator sports, moderate alcoholism, his clubs and the like, or whether he aims at, and achieves, considerable affluence, power, status, economic, political or academic eminence, the plight of all in this era of modern civilization is much the same.

And this plight that man finds himself in, and which he believes has ended any hope for him of physical fitness, and this often before middle-age, indeed, without ever having experienced what it is, even in youth, to be really physically fit, and wholly responsible as a man!

No true, fit and masculine man, surely, is content that any other man fight for him, do his job, or accept the responsibility he should accept. It is even worse to have an attitude of mind that admits of 'saviours' much less someone else 'dying for us'. It is axiomatic, mentally and physically fit men, will do their own living: their own dying: and face up to any deficiencies they may be taxed with. Further, such men never admit, as a finality, the right of any man to absolution, nor will he bend his knee to any anthropological, or anthropomorphic, gods.

An intelligent man will recognise, and admit, the fact that the Universe is governed by Law: Universal, 'Divine' Law, or Natural Law, but to conjure up Vengeful Gods, judgment days, that is an entirely different matter.

CHAPTER SEVEN

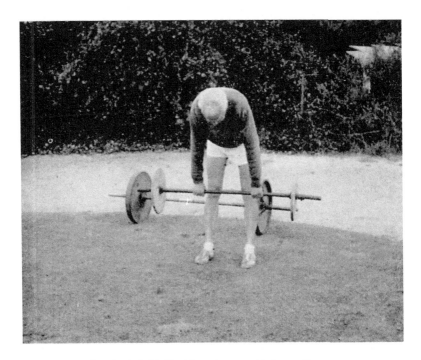

The Rowing Motion. The barbell is lifted from the ground to the position shown. From this position, and without moving the body the weight is pulled up to the chest. This is a good bicep (arm) exercise and places a lot of effort on the abdominals isometrically. The exercise can be done standing when the weight is drawn up to chest level and then lowered to full-arms length.

CHAPTER SEVEN

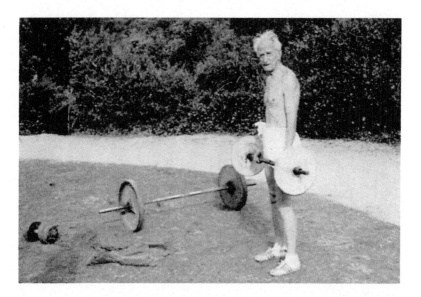

The Cheat Curl. The picture shows the start of the cheat curl. The author is looking towards the camera to see is the picture was taken. Actually the gaze should be straight ahead. From this position the barbell is thrown up to chest level with an outward and upward convulsive movement.

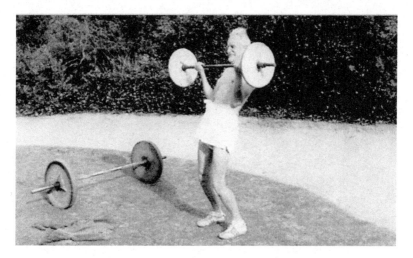

Finishing the Cheat Curl. To heave the weight up the legs have bent as the body dipped a little to assist the upward throw. The object is to bring the whole of the musculature in the movement and not just the arms as when the exercise is done in what is termed the 'Military' Press. I cannot emphasize sufficiently that to get the best all-over exercise results the curl should be performed as a free movement. When done freely and with heavy weights this exercise ranks as the next best all-round exercise to the Dead-lift.

CHAPTER SEVEN

It is far more intelligent to search out the laws of life, and living, and co-ordinate one's life with these laws, simple but adamant as they may be, than to remain ignorant, and expect some 'miracle': some prayer to be answered. Life does not work that way.

It is true psychopathic states can be observed where 'healings' of the physical take place. But for every single cancer that is healed that way, a thousand equally honest citizens die. Is their god so enamoured of psychopaths, favourites, sycophants, even grovellers, and most 'worshippers' come under one of these categories. Where there may be some sympathy for lonely women who turn to such attitudes, surely there is none for men: that is, true, or real, men. That so many men fall short of the requirements to be adjudged 'real' or 'true', is not for this book or discussion.

The fit man is reasonably fearless. Come what may – what financial, political or natural cataclysm overwhelms him he will feel able to wrest a subsistence from his environment. It is because so many otherwise successful men, financially secure, what is termed in the vernacular 'well-oiled', that we see so many terrors: fears and desperations if the nationalistic and ideological movements in the world appear to be jeopardising, much less sweeping away, the investments and sources of income.

The fit man, whilst he will not welcome such losses and changes, will never feel the. desperations and panics that the unfit feel: must feel. This is true since true confidence: integration of the personality, and, under crisis, belief in oneself, arises from the strength and tone of the muscle cells.

I expect it to be repudiated, perhaps as nonsense, when I say, no man unless he can haul a weight that is approaching double his body weight off the ground, or at least, 100 lb over his body weight, is likely to be over-confident in the face of the political and economic changes in the world today, and the possibility of his suffering by, and under, these changes.

Not fit enough to fight, himself, to resist any such changes, he throws all his financial weight and influence into making sure the youth of the country, and who, usually, have little to fight for anyway, especially financially, to do the fighting for him. What a man to accept such an attitude! to bow to such a proposition.

Fitness never betrays: never requires others to do the work we should do. Fitness commands respect: can be relied upon to save us when all else fails: and in the sheer satisfaction derived from living carries with it its own reward. Nothing else quite replaces a high level of physical fitness and muscular strength.

Fitness is the bulwark against the future: it is the real basis of self-respect as it commands, when not the envy, the grudging admiration of others. All things may pass away, but Fitness, and Health, these two, when they abide within you, never desert you.

All others may die, all material things collapse or disappear, but Fitness and Healthy well-being can, and will, be with you always. You may be disappointed: you may hate the task ahead, when your economic life, partly or wholly is destroyed, but with Fitness and Health, like the Phoenix, despite your groans, you will arise to the challenge and, who knows, succeed bigger, and better, than ever before. For the fit – all things are possible.

Summary of Chapter Seven

Do not live in the past: stop imagining: or talking about your wonderful youth. At the time it was not so good – but you have forgotten.

On the other hand, if you are young, or middle-aged, do not sacrifice the present for the, possibly, mythical future.

You may not live to enjoy your retirement, anyway, and if you do, may find you have lost the interest in, and zest for, the things you imagined you would enjoy so much.

Live in the ever-present. Apportion some time: each day, each week, each year, to doing and enjoying something that is disassociated from success, finance, earning and ambition.

What better than Physical Fitness and robust good-health be one of those disinterested pursuits, especially as, when you are older, your high level of physical fitness and health can much better enhance the success you seek, the finance you need, the earnings you would glean, and the ambitions you would achieve.

Too much dedication: too much dying for a cause – any cause. Better to live and work for what you want, whether a cause, a country, or yourself.

It is the 'all-round' life, the many facets of life, that is living. Too much specialization is like 'All work and no play makes Jack a dull boy'.

The zest for living: as for work, is based in some emotion. It can be the emotion that arouses enthusiasm: the desire to live fully, to do something useful, or the emotions that are based in fear, envy, jealousy, even conceit.

Where there is any emotional content, no matter which emotion, the Will is aroused. Without emotion, thinking and intellectually arrived at determinations, seldom provide enough, or continuously aroused, will – to carry through a project.

Heavens, hereafters – 'rewards' and hoping to meet the Saints. All can be, I would say – certainly, are illusions. Such hopes and beliefs can never but be an admission that today is dull and we cannot alter it. Unreal dreams, especially anticipations after death, are substitutions for living satisfactorily today. Only the poor dream of riches: only the sick of being healthy: only the frustrated, those unable to dominate their environment, the incompetents, the unhappy, dream of 'rewards in heaven'. The realist realises his rewards today, and most days. He 'lives': ,the others? they dream!

The education of the mind: the understanding of life: both are essential. Then we are not content to let others fight for us, shoulder our responsibilities, die for us.

CHAPTER SEVEN

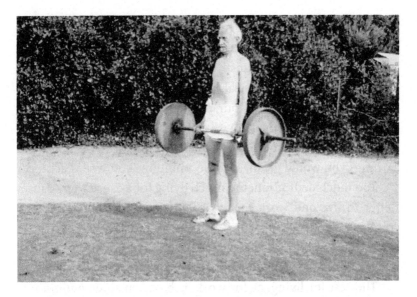

The author commencing a cheat curl with 125 lb (56.8kg) which is 5 lb (2.3kg) more than body-weight. It is considered above average to be strong enough to cheat-curl bodyweight.

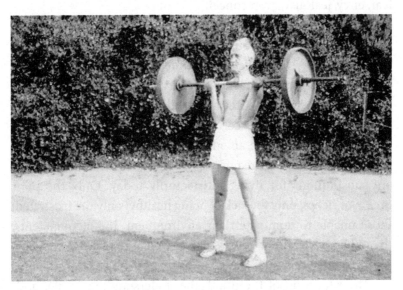

Finish of the cheat curl with a maximum weight. Note how the weight is easily held when the arms rest in close to the body, the legs being well apart, and the hands well apart on the bar. The total position is one of balance, strength and in the absence of strain can even be considered to have beauty.

CHAPTER SEVEN

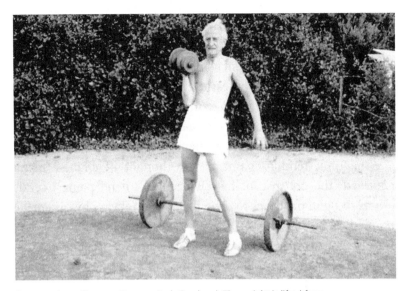

Commencing a One-arm Press, or Push Overhead. The weight is lifted from the ground to a position close to the shoulder, the free arm balancing. Then, with a convulsive movement the weight is thrown, pushed or jerked overhead. This exercise is mostly a back, abdominal and arm strengthener.

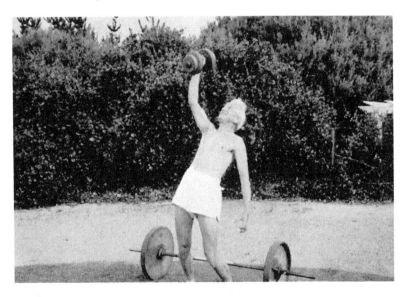

The picture shows the movement just before the completion of the upward throw or jerk. Note that the bent legs and body lean have contributed to the success of the effort. Thus all the musculature is exercised.

CHAPTER SEVEN

The intelligent man will search out the laws of Nature, and not rely upon 'miracles' to supply him with the affluence or health, or happiness, that only intelligent work and understanding can provide.

The Fit are reasonably fearless. In a world where the family fortune can be swept away overnight – the fit man will survive reasonably believing he can cope: can start again. At the worst he knows he will survive, even find happiness.

The unfit tend to panic at the thought of change: being deprived: the collapse of his civilization. So he panics: sends others to fight: proposes to drop his bombs (always by others, be it noted!).

Fitness, real muscular, glandular fitness, that embraces all aspects of life, and women, is the only true bulwark in this changing world.

Most of what happens to us is to test us, and to teach us. What, to the unfit, may be calamity to the fit may be the end of an outworn era, and the commencement of a new era in which we succeed bigger, and better, than ever.

> For the fit – all things are possible.
> Ah, fill the Cup: – What boots it to repeat
> How Time is slipping underneath our Feet:
> Unborn Tomorrow, and dead Yesterday,
> Why fret about them if Today be sweet!

The 37th Stanza of the Rubaiyat of Omar Khayyam.

Chapter Eight

The heart as the key: diet as the chief means: something on the elements of our foods: the importance of vitamins and trace elements.

When all is said and done: when we have examined all the religions: all the sciences: all the philosophies, we come down to one basic fact. It is the heart, and the blood, that are the Key to Life, as we as individuals, if we ever are to enjoy it fully, may experience it.

Like the fuel pump on the automobile, no matter how full of gas the tank may be: how efficient the cylinders, how robust the spark, if the pump fails, that automobile is as dead: it just doesn't move.

Thus the fuel in the tank, the quality of it, and the pump that supplies it to the engine, these two take precedence over all other parts of our automobile.

Even if the spark be weak (the interest in, or desire to live): even if the cylinders be worn, and the pistons slop a bit, even if the gears grind and the 'diff' makes horrible noises, that automobile will move, even if slowly and inefficiently, if the fuel pump is working, and the engine is supplied with suitable fuel. So will man. There is no need to worry about the heart. As I have told you, it has its own mechanism that looks after it, but, and a big 'but', it must be exercised: it must have good fuel (blood) fed to it.

CHAPTER EIGHT

This is so true: so simple: so obvious, that it tends to escape the many, or why the coronaries, heart seizures, high blood-pressures, the strokes, and the sudden deaths!

When these two factors: exercising the heart, and a good blood stream as · uncontaminated as possible, are satisfied, bar an odd contagion, perhaps even then not necessary if we are wise. For instance, the purest blood stream cannot cope with the virulence of syphilis: just as it cannot cope with several other lethal diseases and drugs.

But we are concerned with the normal, not the abnormal condition that the many are never subjected to, anyway.

The pump can be kept efficient and powerful by exercise, but it will break down if the fuel fed into it, and upon which it depends and works, is not as pure as possible, and as free of toxic substance; as possible.

So, given the required amount of exercise, it comes back to the fuel, and the fuel, that is, the blood is exactly what we eat, drink and breathe.

I am certain neither Nature, nor God, never anticipated that man, after fifteen thousand centuries, would ever devise, manufacture and market, the debased and denatured substances that pass for food.

Nor did Nature, or God, ever anticipate that rapacious man, in his selfish desire for self-aggrandisement, would ever have built his food factories, and produced the products of the factories. I feel as equally certain that this is a passing phase, that sufficient intelligent people will realise the tragedy of this food emasculation and, by survival, demand the foods we should eat, in the form the foods should be eaten. The others? they will die, slowly at first, numerically, but with increasing incidence each generation.

Even rats in the laboratory fed only on denatured white flour die quicker than rats left slowly to die from starvation. The almost pure starch of the wheaten flour not only does not sustain life in the rats, but poisons them, since pure, or almost pure starch is a poison.

CHAPTER EIGHT

At this juncture it is interesting to note that human or other animals cannot exist on a diet of fats nor a diet of refined sugars. Just as man cannot exist on alcohol, which is a sugar, or upon food that completely lacks the life principles, and which principles are mainly found in the unadulterated unrefined foods and which include the vitamins and trace elements.

The diet of civilized man in all or most countries (countries like Hunza may be an exception) is so denatured, so poor, that 95 to 99 per cent of all man's ills, and his premature deaths, can be attributed to his food intake.

With a low level of food his natural instincts fall to a low level, and his body will feel but feeble, if any, urges to exercise, even to live as a man should, and would, if his health and zest factors were higher. Our food is made up of protein, carbohydrates (the sugars and starches) fats, indigestible fibres, vitamins and mineral traces.

The tissues of the body are made of protein cells. The growing lad needs more protein than his mature father. Once the body bulk has stopped growing the protein intake should be reduced.

The replacement of the cells, i.e., the body wastage and replacement goes on at a steady rate whether you are a marathon runner, a professional footballer, or an invalid in bed. Effort and energy do not depend upon your protein intake. This may surprise you, since it is not generally known.

In the presence of ample carbohydrates, excess protein foods – the meats, cheese and similar, are passed through the system. In the process much putrefaction may take place.

In the absence of sufficient carbohydrates to provide the energy and warmth needs of the body, any excess protein foods will be availed of. By a most elaborate and long chemical chain the protein elements can be converted into the essential sugars that are used as energy producers.

It is, therefore, a fallacy to believe that, because we have some physical exertion ahead of us, whether it be running a mile or walking ten, that we are best fortifying ourselves with a meat meal. Nothing is further from the truth.

In countries such as Australia and the United States most men eat too much meat. Approximately half a pound of steak, or similar, perhaps three large eggs, or one-quarter pound of cheese''':' anyone of these, not the lot, will provide all the protein necessary in adult life, energetic or not energetic.

It has yet to be proved that excessive protein is not a factor in the growth of a cancer in some types of people since a cancer is merely an excessive growth of cells that have got out of hand and live, as does a mistletoe growth on a tree, until the growth is of such size that the tree wilts and dies.

Cancer, then, is a self-destructive phenomenon since, in destroying the host, and living upon it, whether it be tissue or an organ, it destroys itself. Cancer cells, therefore, appear not to carry with them the 'life' factor, as is inherent in normal cells, and cell replacement. It has yet to be proved that the factor, or one of the factors contributing to the growth of a tumour or cancer is that the diet of the host does not contain sufficient life-principle elements.

Firstly, a cancer can originate from an irritant, external, or introduced into the mouth, throat, windpipe and lungs, or via the mouth, the gullet, or oesophagus, the stomach to the intestines.

Absorbed into the blood stream and distributed thereby, the irritants can be expected to reach every part of the body and all of the organs.

Whilst cancer and the various tumours that maybe, or may not be, malignant, defy the researches as to the actual causes and cures, this much is true: where the body is fed on natural foods, as close to nature as possible, and devoid of the many poisons and irritants that are permitted in processed foods, there is little likelihood of the disease carcinoma in its many forms eventuating in the person who avoids carcinoma excitants, and their number is legion.

CHAPTER EIGHT

It is also true, and proved, that when a person with a tumour, or a cancer, neither of which has progressed to the point of 'no return', and that varies considerably with various persons, and all intake of the normal diet is ceased, and that person fed only on fruit and vegetable juices – and nothing else, a tumour, malignant or not, or a cancerous condition, can clear up.

It is irrational to talk of such improved states as cures. All that has happened is that the irritants that excite the growth of a tumour have been removed from the diet, and the protein that has fed the growth, both have been stopped. The tumour or cancer, where it is not living on the tissue or organ, or cannot draw its sustenance from the tissue or an organ – dies. We call it – cured. Actually, whether in man, the animal or the vegetable Kingdom, where the nutriments are reasonably perfect, and all the other conditions reasonably satisfied, there can be no disease, no blights, nor, generally speaking, any favourable growing or multiplying places for germs, virus parasites, or any other sources of destruction or mutilation.

But the perfect well-being on the physical body depends almost entirely upon the quality of the nourishment that is fed into it.

Where there are deficiencies such as Vitamin deficiencies, or trace element deficiencies, there will be ill-health, malfunction, or a breakdown in the system somewhere.

One of the extraordinary modern day phenomena is that, in research, there is such a lack of recognition as to these factors, although it is well-recognised that, without Vitamin 'C' scurvy ensues, as well as the teeth being affected; that a deficiency in Vitamin B1, causes the disease Beri-beri, and too much lactic acid accumulates in the body: that without Vitamin B2, a person develops Pelagra, of which the symptoms are dermatitis, diarrhoea, even dementia; Rickets occurring with a deficiency of Vitamin D, and in the absence of the required amount of Vitamin E – sterility, either partially or wholly.

If these diseases are caused by a deficiency in the normal diet, how many other diseased conditions, such as hardened arteries (arterio-sclerosis) the various arthritic conditions, lung and other cancers, the rheumatic conditions – are caused, not by deficiencies, but by predisposing elements in the intake. Elements that are introduced by preservatives (all of which are poison and/or irritants): changes in the chemical nature of the foods by factorised (and home) processing, as well as introduced irritants used as colourings and flavourings.

Add to these causes, and commonplace enough in modern civilization, the ease of access, and over-absorption of fats, especially animal fats, of starches and sugars refined to a degree not acceptable to human digestion, the 'dead' foods, such as biscuits, and the addiction to sweets, chocolate, coffee, tea, sugar-drinks, alcohol, and the products of the modern pharmacopoeia, it is not so much that we develop disease conditions, but it is a marvel that the human body can sustain such abuse since for countless thousands of years it knew nothing of these things, nor did it have to cope with them.

Summary of Chapter Eight

The heart, understanding its needs, and supplying these needs, if there is a Key to life – that is it.

If the heart is strong, fed on good blood, then good blood is pumped all over the body. With a constant supply of good blood it is almost impossible to be ill, even contract transmitted diseases. At least, the virulence of contagious diseases will be minimised when the blood is good, and the heart powerful.

In a word, a man with a good heart and good blood will have a chance of surviving under conditions where others die. That is logical enough, surely.

CHAPTER EIGHT

What we eat (diet) what we drink (fluids) and what we breathe (air, contaminated, or otherwise), and nothing else makes our blood, good, bad or indifferent. Nothing else.

Since what the many eat, drink and breathe cannot satisfy the demands as to good blood, then the many become ill, and must die, as they do, prematurely. Do not blame your business, overwork, or your worries as the cause of your ill-health, acidity, ulcer, high blood-pressure, or any other disability from impotence to gall stones. What you 'take-in' is the cause. Nothing else, since if your 'take-in' is perfect, or next to perfect – you won't overwork (you'll see the stupidity of that): you won't worry (you'll know that won't solve anything): and you will be impelled to exercise.

Excess protein, meats etc., over the body's need is cause for danger. You may, or may not be able to cope with the excess. Take no chances, and keep your intake to the minimum suggested in the later tables.

Pure, or almost pure, starches and sugars, of which white flour and white sugar are two prime examples are – in their pure form, poisons. Do not be misled on that one. Reread. Realise what I have said about rats and starch. Realise what a few spoonfuls of sugar would do to a diabetic.

Cancer has causes. Avoid the causes, as you may be avoiding irritants in what you eat and breathe, and obviously – we believe, you will avoid most forms of cancer, at least. Vitamin deficiencies lower the level of health to the point of serious diseases intervening.

Good garden-fresh food will sustain life far better than packeted foods, whilst the 'dead' foods, i.e., those in which the life-principle has been extracted, white flour and refined sugar, being the two most common examples, will not sustain life at all.

Possible causes of cancer could be, not only the irritants, but excessive fats, denatured sugars and starches, and feeding the cancer, excessive proteins.

CHAPTER EIGHT

Whilst these suggestions may be pooh-poohed by some 'authorities' let it be noted, they have no solutions to offer, and die of cancer along with the ordinary 'man in the street' who would not presume to know anything at all – as to causes.

Radium and surgery are poor substitutions for reasonable preventative action. It is a far more sensible attitude to assume that cancer can be prevented, than that cancer can be cured.

I have dealt with cancer. If we are what we eat, then we are, from a point of health, what our blood is, since the blood carries the nutriment to all the organs, and thus maintains them in health. Nothing else does.

So: keep down the Cholesterol level of your blood (no animal fats): reduce your artificial foods, that is your pies, cakes, biscuits, fancy foods, puddings and much else that is accepted as 'good food' to the absolute minimum.

In a word: Eat to live: NOT live to eat.

Chapter Nine

Fats: milk: starches: sugars: salt: vitamins: vegetarianism: raw foods: fluids.

In Nature there are few or no fat animals. It is man who has developed castrated animals that fatten, and provided pastures, free from danger, so that the animals have nothing else to do but eat – and fatten.

All other animals other than man will reject fat as food. It is true some domesticated animals can be conditioned to eat it, but otherwise it can be said – all animals but man reject animal fat.

Animal fat is the fat that is found around various organs, e.g. the kidneys, and plastered upon the muscles, even penetrating the muscles.

Butter and cream are both animal fats.

Whilst some authorities are not convinced, there is sufficient evidence to warrant the statement that the cholesterol level in the blood is definitely influenced by the intake of animal fat.

A person sufficiently interested to wish to keep this level at a minimum will eliminate all animal fat, in whatever form they come, from his diet. In other words, there will be no cooking using dripping, butter or lard, and butter and cream will be omitted entirely from the diet.

Any need at all for animal fat will be adequately met from the flesh foods, beef, mutton, poultry, eggs, and fish that may be normally eaten.

CHAPTER NINE

Apart from the Cholesterol level in the blood, a low animal fat diet will be kindly to the liver and its storage department, the Gall Bladder.

The elimination of the fats will mean no pastries, pies and similar food that, not only being 'dead' foods, are mostly impregnated with animal fat in some form, or another.

Milk is another product of modern civilization. In Nature there are no cows with huge udders, bred and pastured to produce extraordinary quantities of milk with even more extraordinary quantities of butter fat.

The price the cows pay for their artificial evolvement is a number of diseases of which abortion and tuberculosis are common. So much penicillin is pumped into some cows today, here in Australia, at least, that it is readily detected in the milk delivered to consumers, and I know of one case where an adult, allergic to penicillin, and becoming ill, the cause was traced to the milk he consumed. In Nature, no animal, other than man, has access to milk once that animal has been weaned. All the constituents of milk, which are so extolled, are manufactured in the cow from the grass it eats. The cow does not need to eat bone to make bone: eat calcium to make calcium, eat hair to make hair, and so on.

Neither do humans, once weaned, if they live on natural foods, i.e. salad vegetables, fruits, raw and dried, and mostly food that is uncooked and unprocessed, coming from the farm and garden and consumed as found in Nature.

I have found, in my years of association with young athletes, and others, that those youths who have not been properly weaned, and who are still psychologically bound to their mothers, will have an addiction, amounting to a craving, for milk.

I have found that those who are independent, have left home, rejected the over-maternal attitudes of the mother, these young men invariably dislike milk, will only drink it under duress. A high proportion of women, both young and old, dislike milk.

This is because they are not as easily mentally conditioned as the male and, therefore, more natural and instinctive in their tastes and attitudes. Although in this latter regard the customary female addiction to pies, pastry and pimple-producing foods is notorious. However, most women are sensible – instinctive enough, once they realise certain facts, to become the intelligent dietists of the family.

I have already stated, rats in the laboratory fed on denatured white flour alone, die quicker than rats left to die of starvation. The white flour, being almost wholly starch, not only does not sustain life when used exclusively, but acts as a poison. The same can be said of refined white sugar.

It is not impossible that the researchers may find, someday, instead of looking for a virus – as the cause of cancer, they may find that the denatured foods, such as the starches and sugars, carrying with them none of the complete constituents of a natural food, are accepted by the body as an irritant, and that ulcers and tumours are a direct result of the breakdown of the resistance of the organism to these poisons.

Actually there is enough evidence already to support this contention as to Ulcers of the Stomach and the Duodenum.[1]

Dr Berenblum, M.D., M.Sc., a Demonstrator at the Sir William Dunn School of Pathology, Oxford, had this to say: 'The reader may wonder why it took so long to reach this simple truth that *Cancer was not due to bacterial action.*' (The italics are mine.)[2]

Dr Berenblum also remarks, 'Whilst the technicalities of treatment of Cancer are a matter for the Specialist, *the broad principles are very much the concern of the layman.*' (Again, the italics are mine.)

That certain parts of the body, varying quite considerably with different persons, or perhaps not at all in some persons, I give

---

[1] See *Peptic Ulcer* by Dr T. L. Cleave, Formerly Director of Medical Research, R.N. Medical School, Alverstone, England.
[2] Quoted from Science versus Cancer, by Dr Berenblum.

CHAPTER NINE

rise to tumours, does not alter the possibility of why a tumour commences, and grows.

A simple illustration is when we find a Cancer develops upon the face of one person exposed to the sun's rays, and not upon the face of one hundred, or one thousand others. From this observation has come many theories as to why the tumours start in one person and not in another. Cell mutation, inherited characteristics in the Genes, mutated Genes, self-generated virus within the cell, and many more hypotheses and theories.

What is true, apparently, is that a *complete return to Nature's purest nutriments can be a factor in actually curing some Cancers.*[1]

How much more, then, that a strict attention to Nature's diet may be the main preventative, or safeguard, against many forms of cancer. Just as not inhaling tar fumes, certain other chemical irritants, and tobacco smoke can make it almost impossible for anyone to develop lung cancer, no matter what other forms they may become heir to.

Nature, if we are to personalise it, or her, as we do our anthropological gods, hates the artificial: the emasculated: the ultra-refined. Salt: sodium chloride: (NaCl) my dictionary describes it as a necessary ingredient of food for most animals: used by men from time immemorial as a seasoning.

Salt in the form sold and used may yet be found entirely unsuitable for human consumption. Already it is recognised as a factor in hypertension (high blood pressure). It yet may be found to be one of the irritants to the system.

Salt that has been made suitable for human ingestion by metamorphosis may yet be proved to be quite a different chemical when it comes to human nutrition, as is common salt.

Salt, for animals, as for humans, is an easily conditioned

---

[1] *Has Dr Max Gerson a True Cancer Cure.* A Journalist's account of some happenings in a Clinic in New York.

addiction. But that does not prove it is either necessary or good. It is pertinent to observe that, as a horse does not need to have access to salt, to make salt in its own biological laboratory, so neither does man.

Given the essential ingredients, i.e. foods as found in Nature, man does not need to drink hydrochloric acid to make (HCl), nor eat salt to make a natural salt in his body.

Most people, I believe it can be said quite confidently, eat far too much salt with their foods. On a complete food intake (mostly uncooked and unprocessed foods) it has yet to be proved that human beings need to take extra salt because they live in the tropics, or sweat excessively. It is known that the human metabolism can manufacture its own salt if it is supplied with the elements as found in a natural and rational dietary.

Homo sapiens is not a normally evolved vegetarian animal, i.e., herbivorous, any more than man is wholly carnivorous. Man in his pure, natural state, is both. In civilization, he may be attracted to a non-carnivorous diet for humanitarian reasons.

Actually, the HCl (hydrochloric acid) that he secretes in his stomach is there for no other reason than to break down the constituents of flesh foods.

For this reason, since ample HCl abounds in most peoples stomachs it is essential for the acid to have some protein food in each meal, or whenever a person eats. For this reason, it is far more sensible to have a piece of cheese, a cocktail sausage, or a similar protein morsel, when one drinks any other fluid other than pure water.

The introduction of food into the stomach causes the HCl, together with certain pepsins, to be discharged into the stomach. The HCl has an affinity for proteins. Unused, stimulated to excess but no protein in the stomach for it to attach itself to, and digest, it is the reason why so many suffer from acidity: acid eruct ions and even, I have good reason to believe – ulcers.

CHAPTER NINE

Vegetarianism as a humane cult has value. Vegetarianism purely as dietic cult has not. Too many people become cultists of many kinds, mostly to be different. To belong, or give credence to, a minority cult is to engender ego gratification. We are different, so we must be right. My stricture is directed at all cults and cultists. Crankiness, and cultism are not so very much apart, no matter what the cult may be. Intelligent understanding, a realistic attitude based in knowledge will guide one away from pure cultism, or with joining up with other cultists, no matter what the society, group or order may be!

Birds of a feather do collect together. The cry should go out – 'The Good Lord preserve us from the Cultists – in whatever form they appear!'

It is best to take in fluids as a locomotive or an automobile does – at reasonably regular intervals, and only two or three times a day. Fluids are best taken before meals in the case of tea, fruit juice, or water drinking. Alcohol comes under a special dispensation since it is usually not taken as a fluid but as a tranquilliser, of which it is, undoubtedly, the most common and cheapest

It is best, therefore to imbibe alcohol before a meal, together with a little protein food, NOT biscuits, since they are a carbohydrate (starch and/or sugar) alcohol itself is a sugar.

During our meals, one can drink wine, which is a natural product of Nature, even the alcohol content, since there is a little alcohol in the dried fruit of the grape. After all, fermentation is a process in nature, not that I am justifying alcohol, much less alcoholism, but we live in an age where alcohol, in its many forms, is a part of the majority of people's way of life. For this reason it must be discussed as such.

A certain amount of alcohol after a meal will be assimilated with the food. Whilst alcohol may not aid digestion, in small quantities it does not appear to impair digestion. Indeed, the relaxed well-being from its moderate use, in the society we find ourselves in, it may be proved to be an aid since it induces, or should induce relaxation, some peace of mind, and the abandoning of the mind problems that cause tension, and through tension, imperfect digestion, haste and stress.

Therefore, it can be said, on a diet mainly composed of foods as found in Nature: in reasonable proportions, eaten at the most three times daily, certainly never more (so that means, morning and afternoon teas and suppers are eliminated) and preferably, two meals daily, indigestion: cancer of the digestive tract or ulcers, will be nearly, if not absolutely, an impossibility.

Neither beer nor tea or coffee should be drunk with meals or immediately after a meal. I would opine nothing causes more acidity and other digestive disturbances than the universal habit of drinking tea, or coffee, or both, with and after meals.

Beer, especially with food, dilutes the digestive juices and reacts adversely against some. In a word, no fluids with meals other than at most, one glass of water, or the equivalent of wine.

Summary of Chapter Nine

Your need, if any, for animal fats will be met by the normal intake of flesh foods, poultry, eggs and fish. Therefore: no butter or cream, and no lard, dripping or butter in cooking. Use vegetable oils instead.

Except to man, and then, in any quantity only in recent times, even the last hundred years, no animal had access to milk once weaned.

Milk is not good food for humans, once weaned. There are both physiological and psychological, the two being biological, reasons for this statement.

Remember, as you eat, a cancer is often, at least in the beginning, a kind of population explosion of cells, much as we have population explosions, of humans. Keep down the factors that are likely to, firstly, engender that explosion, and later, feed it.

CHAPTER NINE

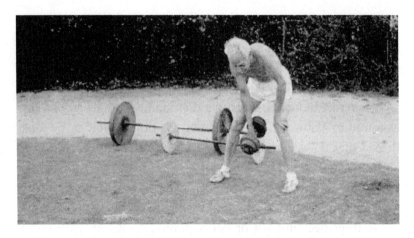

Start of the One-handed Swing. After the weight is lifted clear of the ground it is oscillated between the legs two or three times to gain momentum before being thrown outwards and upwards with as straight an arm as possible. In this exercise all the muscles are exercised especially the back and abdominals. The arms are exercised isometrically when held straight. All the other muscles are exercised isotonically.

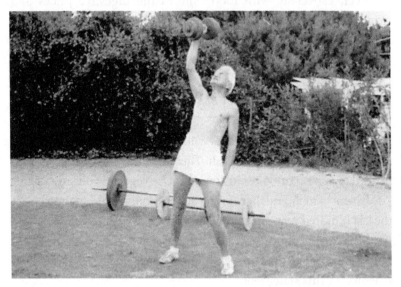

Completion of the One-handed Swing. Because of the weight the author's arm has not straightened. However this is not so important as that a heavy weight is attempted. It cannot be sufficiently emphasized that, except in the case of the deadlift, where some discretion and caution is urged, in all the free exercises the maximum weights reasonably possible should be moved. Otherwise there is little accruement of strength and the exercises are little more beneficial than stretching exercises, and not even then when the exercise is a muscle contracting one such as in curling.

CHAPTER NINE

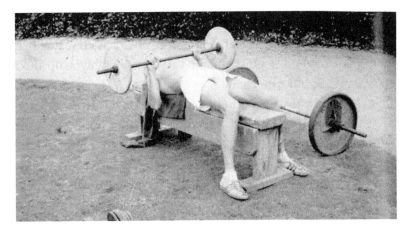

The Bench-press. This exercise mostly benefits the triceps and the pectorals. Of the two, the pectorals, those muscles usually found to be almost non-existent on men who have not exercised vigorously in some form, receive the most benefit. Yet the pectorals strongly support most physical efforts whether it be in vigorous walking and running, wrestling and boxing, and all other sports performed on a high level of efficiency.

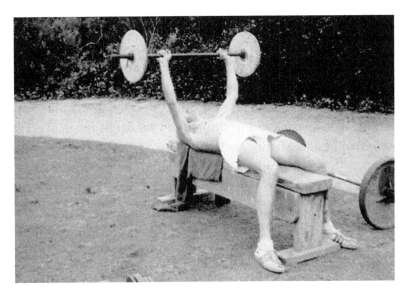

The Bench-press completed. The main disadvantage of this exercise is that it requires an assistant to lift the weight on and off the exercisor. When the exercise is done on the ground the heavy weight may be rolled over the head to the position on the chest.

CHAPTER NINE

Because someone on an identical diet to you does not have a high blood-pressure, an ulcer, or a cancer, do not assume that that diet is normal and good. Humans vary considerably as to their resistances. So: take no chances.

Salt is, mostly, an addiction. The craving is artificial and unjustified in properly prepared foods. Where, however, the natural salts are boiled out, and thrown away, that food will be insipid and a demand will be made for salt. But Sodium Chloride, common salt, is not exactly the same as the mineral salts found in vegetables and meats. Sodium Chloride is a poor substitute and may yet be proved a cause of many ills, not excluding cancer.

If you are a vegetarian be sure you do get sufficient good protein foods in your diet. It is better to be a sensible eater than a famous cultist, whatever the cult may be.

In Nature, there is little that is unique in any group. To return to natural living is not being unique, it is being intelligent. To remain outside what is natural is being, not so much unique, as debased.

Certain things should be accepted as axiomatic. There are little or no animal fats available to man in Nature: certainly not the cream and butter nor the lards, drippings or other sources of the fats used in cooking. If you would be 100 per cent healthy, banish all animal fat, in any form, from your daily food intake. Fat can become an addiction, as is salt.

Banish it, too. You will get sufficient of either in the foods you will eat, even if you move around the world a little, without adding to the quantity by the deliberate use.

Summed up: no butter, no cream: no lards or dripping to be used in cooking (vegetable oils instead) and no salt on the table (and none is necessary in cooking if the food is merely softened and not over-cooked).

Make it a rule: between meals, if the weather is hot – water. Before meals your customary beverages – whether fruit juices, beer, wine, a few whiskies, tea – whatever you drink.

With meals, little or no liquids: positively not tea or coffee with or immediately after a meal. To hell with social customs if your health is at stake.

With meals, perhaps, a small glass of water, or fruit juice, and, if you enjoy it – wine. Certainly not beer with food. Nor after.

Dead foods, that is, foods in which there is no life principle, such as white flour, sugar and the products of both – such foods do not sustain life. Why not eat wholly, or almost wholly, foods that have the life-principle in them.

Foods that 'keep' indefinitely: foods that do not go 'off' in a few days, such as biscuits, some breads, or foods that contain preservatives – these are 'dead' foods: life comes from the life-principle in your foods. From the oxygen in the air and from the life in the foods you eat. If you would survive, fit, healthy, reasonably free of ills and breakdowns of the heart and other bodily organs, make it the rule of your life to – *eat right: drink right: and breathe right.*

Chapter Ten

Certain ideas, axioms and principles need to be understood, and adopted. These factors apply to hunger, weight, and over-feeding.

The scales to weigh the body, stripped, or under the same conditions, are essential: no person, seriously interested in preserving their health and well-being can ignore the necessity for the use of the scales to measure their bodyweight, and in the home.

Scales sufficient for the purpose are not costly. The spring-type may not be accurate, but that is not important. It is not what we may weigh that is important, but how we fluctuate on weight from day to day, and year to year. Here are the facts, at least, as I deduce them.

If a man (or woman) can determine their fit weight registered at 25 years, that weight is their norm for the rest of their life until senility sets in, when previous to dissolution, the weight will tend to steadily fall, as the tissues waste, as they will in the very aged.

Actually, there should be no sudden death, especially while in otherwise apparent health. Man's decease should be a painless process experienced in sheer old age. At the end he will lose interest in the world exterior to himself, and will tend to take to his bed, and refuse food. Both processes make it easier for the life-spirit to cease functioning in that reason. He will become weaker, and will, or should in natural processes, die in his sleep. This is the natural end.

All other are the result of ignorance, stupidity, gluttony, or misadventure.

So, it is important to know what the body-weight was, if fully developed muscularly, and if the life was active. That weight, if known, is the mean for the rest of life.

To achieve this – two important activities are necessary. The first is the control of the appetite; the second is, sufficient exercise to burn up the energy stored, and which, if it is not burnt up, will be stored as fat.

It is a truism, as yet little understood by humanity, if man can overcome his hungers, he overcomes all. The first, perhaps the only hunger to overcome is – belly-hunger. When that simple hunger is understood, and overcome, man, curiously enough, and believe it or not, then, and then only, entirely dominates the self, dominates his environment, bows his knee neither to man or god (he will respect Nature), and realises within his particular orbit, he is master of his destiny. The overcoming of belly-hunger gives all this.

The next step is – each day he weighs himself under the same conditions, and at the same time. It can be on retiring, or on rising. What is important is that the conditions be exactly similar.

With the result on the scales before him each person will know what his food intake should be for that day: whether, if his weight is above the mean, he eats less that day, or if it is below the mean, that he can eat a little more. The regulation of the food intake is precisely similar to the daily input of petrol gas, to the owner of an automobile.

There are certain old wives tales that are dangerous. For sedentary workers, breakfast is NOT the most important meal of the day. It is the least important, and is best not eaten.

Another canard is 'feed the brute'. This is based in two ideas. The first, and most primitive is, that man as the protector and bread-winner have first access to the food available: hence, the idea has arisen over the centuries that, unless he is fed, meaning in modern times – overfed, he cannot work or protect.

The other is the more subtle idea that the way to a man's heart is via his belly and his appetite. So, make a slave of him by providing tempting and special foods and meals. Encourage him to eat more than he needs. He is thus reduced to a degree of slavery, through his belly to you, the cook and housewife. The principle is, better an over-weight lack-lustre husband, even if he die prematurely, than a physically fit, active, rebel who is certain to have a voluptuous eye for another woman, with the reasonable fear that he may clear off with her. Better dead than this happen is the attitude of most wives!

Hunger is natural: appetite is not. It is easy to test whether we eat from hunger or a titivated appetite.

A starving man, or a truly hungry man, will eat ravenously of the plainest of foods until his hunger abates. A man who is not truly hungry will prefer not to eat if the food is too plain, and his palate, dictating his appetite, is not appeased.

When the appetite for food is not debased: when the food eaten is plain and wholesome: when the eater realises the nature and value of the various foods, his enjoyment of simple, plain and natural foods will be enhanced to an extraordinary degree.

Further, the very artificial foods, even foods that can be considered reasonably natural, will be found to be distasteful. With the eating of foods as found in Nature, the appetite for and enjoyment of such artificial foods will be found to have disappeared.

A few simple illustrations will bring this point home.

When one becomes accustomed to eating a good wholemeal loaf of bread, it is found that the white-flour bread is insipid, and the crust rubbery. We find at Portsea, when the Flaked Oatmeal is eaten raw, the taste of the same oatmeal cooked into porridge is insipid.

When one is accustomed to potatoes french-fried in oil, potatoes that are boiled and mashed are almost uneatable, so insipid is the soft mass, especially when butter is beaten in.

When the only biscuits eaten are a wholemeal and oatmeal dried fruit and raisin mixture, the usual biscuits made of refined flours are quite unattractive.

When the body is fed on a salad meal each day, such artificial foods as pies, pastries and cakes, especially soft, iced and cream cakes and confections, become completely distasteful.

The same strictures and attitudes are expected when most, if not all, the various confections, called sweets, puddings, and pastries are eaten.

To the emancipated eater, he not only finds he has lost all taste for denatured and concocted foods, that he is losing nothing, nor suffering any deprivation or hardship, but that he marvels at how others can enjoy such foods, and when he observes them as victims of a false appetite, eating foods irrespective of whether they can possibly be good foods, but from the pleasure the depraved palate gets – then that observed eater falls by just that much in the respect that he otherwise may enjoy.

Despite what gifts, brilliance of mind, wealth or position, a person who gives evidence of being an alcoholic, a drug addict, a glutton, or non-discriminating in the matter of intelligent eating and drinking, such a person must fall by just that much in the respect of others not so addicted. Often the sight of others eating and drinking is repulsive, and arouses, not even sympathy, much less respect, but revulsion.

The intelligent person who controls as much as is reasonably possible, not only his weight, his gluttony, his drinking habits, but his destiny, will be found to be the person mostly envied and respected.

He will be found to be the type of person who has a mind of his own: who is not easily dominated by men or women: who will not readily capitulate, and will be recognised as one who 'paddles their own canoe'.

To recapitulate: He who overcomes belly-hunger is he who overcomes all.

CHAPTER TEN

Summary of Chapter Ten

Own your own scales: if you want absolute accuracy buy a beam scale. Otherwise, the cheap form of spring scale are quite efficient since their accuracy can be checked. To do this, weigh yourself clothed, or unclothed, then proceed without any variation at all, such as eating or evacuating, and weigh upon the check scale. Any error will be evident.

The error can be allowed for on your 'home' scales. However, it is the variation in your weight from day to day that is important, and later, vital.

Remember: it is rare to see a grossly over-weight man over 60 years of age: and as rare to see an over-weight man, at all, over 80.

If you pinch the loose flesh on your abdomen between your thumb and forefinger, and you find you have more than half an inch of fat in that area, consider yourself several pounds overweight. You won't die because of it, but you will be wise not to let your girth grow.

Do not look upon death as 'chance': something that you have no control over. That attitude is one of the most unintelligent sophistries ever promulgated by ignorant men.

The appetite MUST be controlled, whether it be for food, alcohol or drugs. If you would eat well you must be reconciled to exercise hard.

Unused calories, where the digestion is good, are stored as fat. So: either burn up your calories by hard, sweating exercise, or cut down on them.

Eating various foods because they are 'nice', especially soft foods, cakes, pies and pastries, are evidence of a certain juvenile state that should pass away with maturity and adulthood.

All your life your weight should not exceed your fit and fully-muscular development, at least, under so. Ageing is no reason for weighing more. There is no virtue in portliness.

Clothed bulk may look impressive: naked bulkiness is certainly repulsive. And finally, and to repeat: 'When we overcome belly-hunger, we overcome all!'

Chapter Eleven

On exercise: why it is essential to exercise: man's main weakness: the two chief exercises: the degree of exertion in walking and running.

I have said, man has existed in some form for nearly two million years. Until the last few ticks on the time clock he just had to exercise, or stay put.

Walking was the chief exercise. Many men not only walked distances of ten miles but carried heavy loads of provisions. To walk 30 and 40 miles in a day was common place.

Even with the advent of horses to ride, and to pull carts, considerable exercise was involved. Often the horse had to be caught. It required exertion many men today would be incapable of, to mount a horse, even to clamber up into a cart.

The jolting received, whether riding a horse, or sitting in a coach or dray, because of the condition of the roads, the jolting caused a certain amount of movement, even if not exercise, in the strict sense.

Then everything had to be lifted. Everything that had to be moved from soil on the shovel, to timber, bricks, everything – all meant back-bending, and powerful arms and shoulders.

In a short 50 years all has been changed.

I have already said, no organism can have its environmental

factors markedly altered without grave risk to its survival. Modern man has largely placed himself in the category of the doomed, at least, the partly doomed.

In its earliest evolvement the creature that man ascended from spent much, if not all of its time, on all fours. To this day a blind baby, not lifted to its feet and taught to balance and walk, will never walk as a biped.

The pelvis and arrangement of the limbs make it easier, and more restful, to be on all fours. The constant lifting and pulling kept the shoulders forward and the spine straighter than we find today.

Because most men no longer bend and lift the spinal column is not exercised. Two conditions hardly known, or not known at all, are now commonplace. The conditions are backaches, and slipped discs.

Both conditions are painful. They are one of the chief causes of emotionally unsatisfied wives.

Walking, and running, are both as natural and necessary for physical fitness as sitting and lying.

It is a truism that, for countless generations man, because of his exertions, sweated most days. Therefore, sweating from exercise, most days, can be considered an essential part of his daily life and routine. Unless it is from the heat of the day, or their environment, most men no longer sweat, or are submitted to exertion violent enough to cause them to sweat. Man is becoming, and will increasingly become, weak and effete. Faced with an early loss of his procreative powers, he will have little reasonable chance of attaining even 70 years, and because of that one factor alone, absence of sweating exercise!

The two main exercises, and upon which all else hangs, i.e. the efficiency of the lungs and heart, the strong back, a generally and reasonably muscled upper body and arms, and the most vital of all, hard powerful abdominals, and legs that retain the appearance, and strength, of what legs should be are:

CHAPTER ELEVEN

1. Pedestrianism, which includes both walking and running.
2. Dead Lifting, to which we can add curling, although that is not absolutely essential.

We shall deal with pedestrianism.

Every man should average, as a minimum, two miles per day. This requires an expenditure of time of 30 minutes.

His walking should be vigorous, and his object to reduce the time occupied. Two miles ambling in 20 minutes should be within the scope of most.

It is not essential that a strict daily regime be observed but his fifteen or so miles per week should not be crowded into an effort on one day, by a long walk in the weekend. He should have two or three mile walks during the week, every week.

It is less than fifty years ago that most men achieved this standard, walking to the transport of those days. Today many men walk only the few yards to their car. They may walk in this manner, a mile or two each week, but they never sweat nor become tired from their exercise. Both sweating and some tiredness are essential.

They may walk three or four miles playing golf in the weekend, but the nature of that exercise, whilst tiring, is still not as vigorous as it should be.

The solution is easy. Our fit man programmes his life to include his walk! He can walk vigorously to and from transport. He can park his car some distance from his destination: he can make provision to walk of an evening, at least, twice during the week.

If he is not too far gone physically, and I personally know the Managing Director of a large business who runs most days: whilst a Governor-General of Australia to the end of his days, kept up his daily run at least into his eighties. A famous Australian Surgeon did likewise. These typify persons who preferred to run.

CHAPTER ELEVEN

Actually: if one is not too decrepit: if the blood pressure is not too high: and the old body and legs can be goaded to the task, running is far more exhilarating: far more beneficial: and saves far more time.

Again, the running does not need to be done daily, but the minimum should be three times a week. The objective is to persist until one mile can be reasonably covered without resting, exhaustion or collapse! It is best to start this way: In the early morning, or before retiring, the 'performer' gets into some clothing reminiscent of his youth. An old football jersey or similar, an old pair of slacks, a broken-in pair of tennis shoes, with socks, and away he goes.

He can commence (when not observed by critical, cynical or amused neighbours) by jog-trotting for, perhaps, 100 yards. If this causes some puffing, even a slight palpitation he can walk to recover. When the breathing is normal he will essay the jog again. According to his degree of fitness (or unfitness) he will essay a quarter mile, or the full mile, or some intermediate distance.

For a start it is best to travel round the local streets, or a nearby park, or sports oval. It is a mistake to head away and then find, when tired or winded, that one has to cover the distance to return.

In the beginning it must be – hasten slowly. But every effort should be made to extend the effort, i.e., the distance jogged, until eventually, the mile can be covered. The next step will be to try and increase the speed of the effort. This can be done by quite a burst for one hundred yards, then a jog, even a walk, until recovered, until it is found that the mile can be covered at quite a reasonable speed.

Incidentally, such efforts can become very challenging: therefore, quite interesting. And the desire to improve and excel can be quite a determinant as to the other factors of fitness and health, the watchfulness as to eating and drinking.

For a commencement, a man who can walk a mile in 20 minutes should be able to jog the mile under 15 minutes.

When really fit and able to run with some speed, the mile could be covered in ten minutes for any fit man of 40 years of age. Those with some aptitude, considerably faster, perhaps.

But the speed is not important. It is the effort that is important, and the effort is related to the breathing and the sweating induced.

Whether walking, or running, every effort, at first consciously, must be made to keep the movements fluid, the arms rising and falling, as well as swinging forwards and across the body.

These simple movements are necessary if the lungs are to be fully filled and completely emptied, as we walk or run.

Mostly, civilized man, including most athletes it is interesting to observe, would appear to have lost the natural ability to fill and empty the lungs – and it is this lost natural capacity to breathe deeply and fully that prevents most efforts being considerably better than they are found to be.

It is the deep and full breathing that cleans out the lower lobes of the lungs, sets the heart's rhythm, and supplies the much needed oxygen.

Indeed, deep and full respiration should be sought and practised until it is habitual, even when sleeping. After attention to diet, this could be the greatest single factor in healthy longevity.

If we assume a daily run of a mile that means six or seven miles for the week. The enthusiast will soon want to exceed this figure. By running a mile every other day, rather than too strict a daily regime and a good try-out of three miles one morning in the weekend – he will equate his weekly task.

To improve on his mileage he could build up until a weekly run of five miles, even ten, is not beyond his powers, supported by a few runs of a mile or so daily, or two or three times in the week.

It will soon be found that the heart will strengthen and the normal resting pulse rate will be found to be lower than the customary 72 to 80 beats per minute, and which is mostly found in men over 40 years of age, even those who believe themselves to be reasonably fit.

However, before any athletic extravaganza a wise man will have his blood-pressure tested by a medico. If the norm is accepted at 80/120 it is not anything to worry about if the upper reading is as high as 140. Actually, it is the differential that is, also, important.

Another test of the heart's efficiency and the efficiency of the whole bodily organism, is the speed at which the pulse rate drops. With a young well-trained athlete it is possible to drive the pulse up in the order of 200 beats per minute.

For the older man with a normal, even for his age permitting a little latitude, pulse rate, it is quite permissible to drive the pulse rate, by some hard running effort, to the order of 130, even 140 beats per minute.

However, to repeat, before any of such efforts, the wise man will have the medico listen via the Stethoscope to the beating of the heart, and test for any unusual sounds in the lungs.

Receiving the 'all-clear' for the heart, lungs and blood-pressure, there is little or no danger from even what may be considered – extreme exertion. When the three main factors are satisfied, viz., heart, lungs and blood-pressure, overdoing it (which is unwise) will cause dizziness, a sick-feeling in the stomach and extreme shortness of wind. Short of these three warnings, in the matter of effort, it is purely an individual matter, one man absorbing an effort much easier than another.

So, it is a matter of moderation in all things. But it is normal to test oneself out, perhaps, once a week. Man, normally, and by nature, is a competitive animal. It is good to test oneself out, firstly, against one's own personal best, then later, against the best of another man.

But killing oneself to prove oneself: or just to best another, is hardly the action of an intelligent adult. The instincts usually warn us to desist long before there is any real danger.

After all there are no brave men, no heroes – as there are no rich men – in cemeteries, only the deceased!

CHAPTER ELEVEN

Summary of Chapter Eleven

Walking, and running, are the two basic primary and elementary movements of man.

Running is as natural as eating: it should be considered an essential form of movement, and not merely a sport for the young or an eccentricity for the older man.

For countless ages man moved by no other means walking and running. In the last generation, or two, he has increasingly abandoned both.

The heart can never be as strong and fit without this primitive pedestrianism as it normally should be. Calisthenics or any similar form of exercise, does little or nothing to strengthen the heart.

Exercising the heart only occurs when the walking or running is done to the point of sweating and deep breathing. Slow walking is much more a mental relaxation than a heart strengthener.

If you prefer walking, make it hard, and average two miles per day, or missing some days, 15 miles per week.

If you would avoid being dubbed a crank, an exhibitionist, or an eccentric, do your exercising in the early morning or the evening. The early morning especially is delightful.

There is no need to dress up. Any old woollen garment, an old pair of slacks (or shorts), old tennis shoes and socks is all that is required. Certainly not jock straps or suspensories. They are completely outmoded. Not only useless but restricting.

To run: commence jogging in easy stages, say 100 yards, rest or walk until recovered, and jog or run another 100. Do this, unless very weak, until the total distance covered is one mile.

The aim is to lengthen the distances run and to shorten the distances rested and walked until the mile can be covered without walking, or resting at all.

Having run a mile, no matter how slowly, the next aim is to try and improve the speed. A trial once a week is interesting.

CHAPTER ELEVEN

By now the business of fitness has become an interesting, even an absorbing, game.

For the relatively unfit and untrained, at least for some years, a mile covered in ten minutes can be considered good over 40 years of age. A mile in eight minutes is excellent, whilst a mile in six minutes is rare.[1]

The author at 20 years of age was able to run a mile in 4:30 with little training, certainly not an average of five miles training per week.

At 40 years of age he couldn't run a mile at all. His ill health and unfitness made the effort of running a ¼ mile as much as could be managed at the slowest jogs. Running a total of 1,300 miles in the three years after 48 years of age, he managed to run several one mile races, each under five minutes. In his sixties his best time for the mile was 5:32, and on his 70th birthday, he ran a mile in 6:36. The author does not run daily, some weeks, not two miles for the week because of other pressing duties and activities.

Make sure, in all walking and running, that the arms move freely, up and down as well as forward and across, and that the abdominals work, otherwise there will be no full and deep breathing.

It is not necessary to exercise daily, but at least three times per week is called for. If your resting pulse rate is under 80 beats per minute you should be fit enough to start. Check on this and get your medical man to listen to your heart and lungs for irregularities, also test your blood-pressure. He is sure to urge caution if you tell him what you are about to do.

However, never overdo it. Watch for the symptoms of nausea, dizziness or difficulty in breathing. It is easy to become over-enthusiastic.

Be wise: be sensible: and – live!

---

1 N.B. These figures apply to the ordinary man who has not trained, or kept up his training for athletics or other vigorous sports.

Chapter Twelve

> *After energetic walking, or steady running, the next important exercises are those that strengthen, and maintain the tone of the back and abdominal muscles*

Apart from the muscular condition of the shoulder, back and abdominal group of muscles, all essential for the well-being, physical fitness and masculine assertiveness of the adult male animal, it is not sufficiently recognised that the internal organs and glands take their tone from the muscles contiguous to them.

It can be considered axiomatic if a man has powerful abdominals, no excess belly fat, and his back and the muscles associated with the lower back in particular, are all strong and well-developed that he will have powerful and explosive intestines, or lower bowel, and will be free of difficulties in urination. He will normally be sexually vigorous.

Just as vigorous walking with a powerful and full arm action will develop the shoulder group and pectorals, so by association, that man will have a good, powerful, and certain other factors being satisfied, disease-free heart.

It is trite to remark that the other factors, a fat-free diet, a natural food intake, a moderate alcohol consumption, if any, and a nicotine-free inhalation of air, will almost certainly be observed if the person is really interested in his physical well-being, and feels the need for, the benefit of, and a certain exhilaration for life and living.

Actually, for such a man his problem will be feeling he is held captive by his work, and the conditions and the form, and the mores, of the civilization in which he finds himself.

For instance, he may find himself, and feel himself, fit enough to want to travel: to climb: to experience: to explore, and worst of all, enjoy the society of the many women he may encounter.

Thus his physical fitness may well be offset by certain frustrations rather than inhibitions. But it is to be remembered that there is a price to be paid for everything – every advantage in life, as a price is paid, eventually, for every weakness, every excess, every dissipation, every ignorance. Never was it more true, in the matter of physical health and well-being, and I am not concerned, at the moment, with the morality of any act – that 'virtue hath its own reward'.

After all, virtue can mean being thoughtful: acting intelligently: and realising that, in the end, Nature's Laws cannot be bucked. It is even better, although I am stating something now, rather than advocating a course of action, that it is far better to buck the canons of society than develop a neurosis: acquire a fixation about altering something unalterable, or become an alcoholic – the three main outlets for many men in modern society.

However, the price to be paid in fitness, the effort required to be fit, is repaid a hundredfold to the man who would live: the man who will not turn away from the present limitations, or the apparent hopelessness of his frustrations.

It is in this field that miracles do occur; so, without more ado: to our exercises.

The simplest, and probably as efficacious, even if not as satisfying as some other exercises, is the SIT-UP.

This exercise requires no apparatus: can be done anywhere

where there is a six feet space to lie down and something to put the feet under. Proceed as follows:

Choose a place where, lying flat upon one's back, the feet can be placed under a wardrobe, desk, or other piece of furniture. This is to prevent the feet rising when the body is eventually raised. If some such furniture is not available then a loose strap should be fixed to the bottom of the door, or wall, about eight inches from the floor. The strap needs to be at least 15 inches long, and so loosely fixed that both feet are easily placed behind it. It also needs to be sufficiently strong to withstand a pressure, possibly as high as 100 lb.

The 'victim' of the 'torture' to come places both hands behind his head. Using his hands by pressing on his head he aids his abdominal muscles, to bring the trunk upright into a sitting position. To do this he will find that his knees want to bend until, perhaps, they are raised, some six or eight inches from the floor. This is quite okay. It keeps the whole exercise fluid, is more natural, and permits the head to be brought forward, if not in the beginning, later, to a position between the knees.

In doing the above it will be noticed how a pressure is put upon the restraining furniture or strap that holds the feet down. This, in itself, is good, since it is a form of isometric exercise that strengthens the ankles and the thighs especially.

If you are reasonably fit you will have little difficulty in doing this exercise ten times. Whether it is ten times or one hundred a stage is soon reached where an acute pain is felt across the abdomen in the region of the navel. This is normal and indicates that the exercise has reached a point where it is doing you good.

However, do not be too venturesome, or courageous, at the beginning. Desist when this pain is felt. To persist in the early stages will mean you will feel very stiff and sore in that region, although I doubt if any other harm can accrue.

Sit-ups can be done daily, or several times in the day. At home, at work, anywhere at all. They can be continued until one hundred can be done without resting. However, a daily dozen will keep the abdominals fit. The hundred is for the enthusiast.

If it so happens that the beginner has not sufficient strength to do even one sit-up, he can fix a rope or strap to a ring in the wall at a height of about three feet from floor level. A stout rope is attached and is used by the exerciser to help pull himself from the prone to the sitting position. When sufficient abdominal strength has been gained the rope can be discarded.

When one hundred consecutive sit-ups have been accomplished, the exerciser is ready to do his sit-up on an inclined board. This requires some apparatus. A fixed height board can be provided, or a board made so that it can be fixed to rails placed at various heights. The greater the elevation of the feet and the lower the head, the more strenuous the exercise.

Whilst very strong athletes can do repetitive sit-ups on an inclination as great as 90 degrees – the body being at right angles to the floor – such efforts are usually beyond the scope of the man over 40 years of age.

Efforts against the stopwatch can be done competitively. These competitions can be on the floor level or upon the Inclined board. Athletes at Portsea have completed one thousand sit-ups from the horizontal plane (lying upon the board) in one continuous effort. The author achieved one hundred repetitions as routine, preferring to work on the inclined board, where, in professional exhibitions a best of ten seconds for ten sit-ups has been achieved. The Inclined Board used in television and other demonstrations, has an inclination of 20 degrees, the feet end of the board which is five feet six inches long, being two feet above the horizontal or floor level. (See picture.)

If this exercise is approached with reasonable caution, little or no harm can accrue. Even with over-enthusiasm nothing worse than a feeling of soreness and stiffness of the abdominal muscles

CHAPTER TWELVE

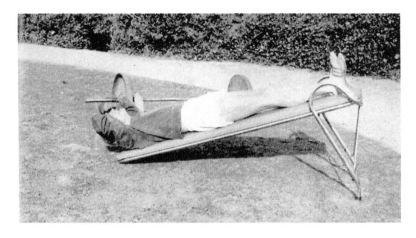

The Sit-up using an Inclined Board. Such a board can be fixed to a rack on a wall. On an inclined board the exercise requires much more strength. The feet require to be held under a strap to perform the exercise at all.

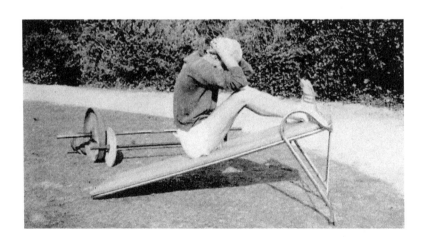

The completion of the Sit-up on the Inclined Board. Other than the body being tilted the exercise is precisely the same as the prone-on-the-ground Sit-up. The head should finish between the knees which are drawn up to meet the head. Working on the Inclined Board as shown the author has achieved ten repetitions in ten seconds.

CHAPTER TWELVE

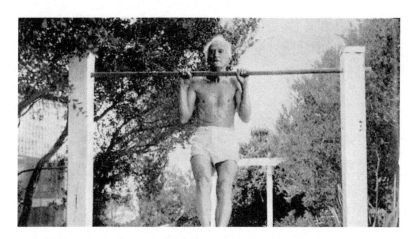

Another good exercise that requires apparatus – The Chin on the Horizontal Bar. Whilst the arms receive all the isotonic benefit the abdominals and the legs receive some benefit isometrically. A horizontal bar, and a barbell should be considered part of the equipment in every household.

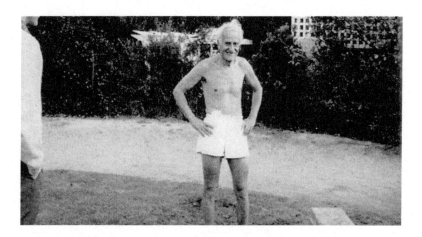

The author, in his seventy-second year, healthily tired, relaxed and happy after an exercise session. Note: The young man in this picture, David Pottage, lives with the author and his wife as part of his physical education. Aged now sixteen years, at fourteen years of age he achieved one thousand sit-ups without resting or stopping.

should occur. It is normal and natural for a human being to raise himself in this position. Where an exercise is normal and natural there is little risk of strain, rupture or any other disability other than soreness until the exerciser becomes adapted to the work.

Nevertheless, the sit-up is as essential as is walking: and working on the inclined board as normal as running.

The ability to walk fast, and run when required to do so, together with the sit-up can be considered the basic evidence of masculine strength and fitness. Some ability in all three suggest a physical well-being that, being normal, means that the individual will have confidence in himself: he will know, and feel himself, to be a 'man'.

Summary of Chapter Twelve

After walking and running which are the best exercises for the heart as a muscle (swimming and skating are both beneficial, it is needless to remark), exercises that benefit the back and abdominal muscles are next in importance. The simplest form of exercise to benefit the back and stomach is the sit-up.

It is best, I would say – essential, that the feet be held down by a strap on the wall, or being placed under a heavy article of furniture.

For the feet to be firmly held brings in isometric exercising of the legs themselves. Thus a two-fold beneficial result is achieved.

To begin, place the hands behind the head and help the body to rise by pulling or forcing the head, upwards and forwards until it reaches a position between the knees.

The knees should bend and come up to meet the head. Because of these movements it is more comfortable to rest the buttocks on a cushion.

If the sit-up is beyond you due to lack of strength or general unfitness, commence by fixing a rope to a wall and assisting the

CHAPTER TWELVE

body to a vertical position by pulling on the rope.

Ten 'reps' of the sit-up exercise, daily, will keep the abdominals in good tone. This good tone reflects by association upon the organs and glands of the abdominal cavity.

One hundred 'reps' can be considered in the championship class. But there is no sense in overdoing any exercise until one is strong enough to do the exercise with reasonable, and NOT exhaustive ability.

An Inclined Sit-up Board can be used. Exercising on an angle where the feet are higher than the head when the body lies prone is like running is to walking: the benefit is cut down in time, although the effort is harder. Ten to 20 sit-ups on an inclination of 45 degrees can be considered the equivalent of one hundred sit-ups done from the horizontal plane, i.e., lying on the floor.

Again the axiom must be: 'Hasten Slowly'. 'Feel' your way to Fitness, rather than strain yourself seeking it.

Chapter Thirteen

Dead-Lifting: The Basic and Best Exercise, and most natural of all Exercises using apparatus.

If there is one movement basic in man, other than perambulation, it will be lifting.

Man would never have survived if, after having walked to an object, he had been unable to lift, if the lifting was needful for his purposes.

To survive man has needed the strength to bend down and hoist from the earth the larger animals that he would have transported to his caves, and for his own sustenance, as well as the sustenance of the women and children. The caves in which prehistoric man sheltered have been found to contain the bones of the many animals that primitive man consumed for food.

Later, he needed to bend, lift and haul stones and trees to make huts and palisades. Until a century ago all moving of heavy articles was done manually. In many countries, to this day, all labouring work is performed manually.

It is interesting at this juncture to remember that less than the century ago – indeed, within my own recollection – there was no incidence of slipped discs, and back-ills were mostly unknown. Other than the sedentary occupation of the many, and the increasing consumption of denatured food-stuffs, what other factor

CHAPTER THIRTEEN

can be deduced as the cause of man's bark troubles, and corpulence.

The answer must be, the cessation of lifting, even in its simplest form, stooping to pick up objects, and lifting even a spadeful of soil. What then can modern man do to rectify this condition, something which was a part of his very existence for nearly two million years and which in the last tick of the time clock, he has found a machine and which he has assumed has obviated the necessity for exerting himself, even in the slightest, in this way.

It is not suggested that, to make good this deficiency, that the man who resides in a large city attempts to find large stones and tree-trunks to move around, nor can he expect to carry a carcass from the abattoirs to his home. Such ideas are, obviously, absurd.

On the other hand, if he is going to remain a strong human, fully functioning, and able to rally to the demands that may be made upon him, he must do something to compensate for the change in his environment and accept the conditions of his survival.

The answer is – in exercising with the barbell. This comparatively recent contrivance simulates the conditions under which man lived, and still must live.

Just as he is find finding that to have the wealth that makes it unnecessary for him to walk, lift or move his musculature at all other than to lift a knife and fork, a glass, and then to swallow – that he soon develops a physical state that engenders heart, digestive, intestinal, bladder and other breakdowns. He finds that he becomes over-weight, impotent, and with an expectation of life far short of the three-score years and ten.

It is not suggested that to buy a barbell is the entire answer. It is suggested that to recognise a few simple facts, and to act upon this recognition, can revolutionise the life of most, if not all, men.

Today, the barbell in the home is a must. Let us trace the domicile of man over the last few centuries in Europe.

Only 100 years ago he was lucky to have the various rooms looked upon, not only as necessary, but normal, today. His

CHAPTER THIRTEEN

kitchen was his living-room. He probably had no separate room as a bathroom. Today, other than the indigent poor, a family man expects to have a living-room, as distinct from his cooking area. He expects to have a bathroom, and, if his house is large, two or more. He expects to have separate bedrooms, at least separating the sexes: a Sun-room, a study, a Nursery and toilet facilities, all under the same roof. Even his automobile is often garaged under the same roof. But few men have realised the importance of the 'Home Gym': that room, or area, devoted to his fitness, his exercises, and something enjoyed by the whole family.

This book is not the place to deal with all the apparatus and equipment that could be found in the complete home gymnasium. It will suffice to bring under notice the importance of the barbell and the two or three essential exercises if man is to survive, in perpetuity, as a species upon the Earth.

The modern barbell is a vastly different piece of apparatus to the old dumb-bells, with their fixed weights, and unwieldy shapes. Today, the nickel, or chrome-plated bar, the disc shaped weights, usually painted red, are not only a joy to look at, but a pleasure to handle and lift. In addition, with the variety of weight in the discs varying from 1 ¼ lb. to 50 and 60 lb, any weight at all can be quickly assembled for any exercise, and to meet the needs from the youngest to the strongest in the family.

In a modern home, no family should be without a barbell, an inclined board, a skipping rope, or two, and the desire – indeed, a pressing urge to go out and run a mile or so. Back to the basic exercise, the King of all Lifts, the Dead-Lift. So-called because, to drag a weight off the earth, little or no technique is necessary. One is either strong enough to lift a given weight, or one is not. The weight, being inert, is called 'dead'.

In the beginning, certain rules need to be observed. Firstly, with little or no experience of lifting weights, no attempt should be made to lift a weight more than half of the lifter's body-weight.

CHAPTER THIRTEEN

We will assume the lifter has a bodyweight of 160 lb., he can load the barbell so that the total weight, which includes the bar itself – usually in the order of 25 lb. – is 80 lb.

He now lifts that weight in the manner to be described. Firstly, he approaches the barbell and stands facing it with his feet under the bar, not the whole of his feet, of course, but the instep and toes. Then he lowers his body to seize the bar by bending his legs. In doing this his shins will contact the bar itself, his knees protruding over and beyond the bar.

In this position the lifter's body should be as erect as possible, the back flat and the shoulders some 18 inches higher than the buttocks. On no account should the lifter bend over the bar with a curved back and shoulders down to the level of the buttocks.

The best grip is one hand over and the other under (see close up photo). The actual moving of the weight is done by straightening the legs, resisting the tendency of the body to bend over, and finding as the legs straighten, the barbell passes the knees that protruded over it.

When the legs are straightened the movement of the body is carried on until it is perfectly upright. Then the shoulders are moved backwards until the shoulder-blades meet at the back. The weight is then lowered to the ground or floor, by bending over a little, and the legs bending.

It is important to know, and to realise fully, that in dead-lifting, *until the lifter's organism is fully strengthened*, and only after much practice (certainly months for a younger man, and possibly years for a man aged over 40 years, and unaccustomed to such exercises), he can strain various parts of his organism.

Therefore, heroic attitudes, bravado and foolishness cannot be tolerated. If an exerciser finds he lifts half his body-weight with ease, he can proceed to do as many as five (5) repetitions. After a week or two he can move to ten (10) repetitions. When he can do ten repetitions as routine, and without any exertion, he can add five pound, perhaps ten pounds, to each end of the barbell, and go back to five repetitions with the new weight.

For health and fitness little or nothing else is required. The whole operation takes but the same time usually spent in shaving, but can be of inestimable benefit.

As his strength improves so he can add more weight working on his five and ten 'rep' schedule until some day he may be able to lift, in one lift, even double his body-weight.

However, this feat is for the extra strong and no sensible man will attempt, or expect to perform the feat, without some years of lifting and much experience and knowledge.

The ordinary run of citizens over 40 years of age can be well-pleased if they are able to heave their body-weight off the earth in a single dead-lift, and if they can manage five or ten 'reps', without any exhaustion other than a slightly quickened breathing when the 'reps' have been completed – he can deem himself – 'strong', and certainly above normal for his age, and in any society.

Now for a few 'Don'ts', and warnings.

Never lift within two hours of a hearty meal, or any meal for that matter. If one feels a need to do so, empty the bladder before lifting. Remember: to benefit safely from this exercise you lift on your *strength*, never on your *will*. Even when lifting over body-weight, the lift must be done by a conscious delivering of strength, never by calling up the will: the do or die effort.

As is so with most things in life, the best things carry with them the most responsibilities, and dangers. Dead-lifting is no exception. If it is necessary for the back to bend over from the erect position, then that weight is too heavy, and any attempt to lift it abandoned.

Otherwise there are no real risks of strains or ruptures. Follow the suggestions closely: cease if there is the slightest sign of heart palpitation, or stertorous breathing. And above all, be conscious of, and watch for, the slightest feeling of strain in the groin area extending from the lowest part of the abdomen upwards and to the side.

The advantages to be derived may well out-weigh any risks of injury. The advantages are: a feeling of well-being, of being strong and powerful: of confidence in oneself as an adult in competition with his fellow-man: a belief in one's own virility whatever that normal standard may be, and which varies with all men.

Finally, I do not believe that dead-lifting actually 'exercises' the heart. The heart needs to be exercised and strengthened by much longer and steadier periods of exercise. What is true, is that the heart responds to the call made upon it by the extremely strenuous nature of the exercise of dead – lifting. If it is strong, exercised, and not expected to function on toxic blood, all can be well: all *will* be well.

And last of all, in these days of accidents and emergencies on the world's highways, how advantageous, how egogratifying, if a strong man is wanted to help lift an automobile off an injured person, or child, and one can respond to the call without undue risk. How unmasculine to have to refrain because of one's accepted weakness, or how foolish to attempt to help when not fitted to do so.

Summary of Chapter Thirteen

Dead-lifting, that is, heaving heavy articles whatever their nature may be off the earth, must be considered a primary physical function of *homo sapiens*.

Domestic, and modern society, makes it somewhat impossible for man to lift and hunt as did his ancestors from time immemorial to quite recent times.

The scientific barbell has replaced rocks and tree trunks: lifting and hurling his enemies and shouldering the carcasses of animals.

CHAPTER THIRTEEN

In a society where most members can afford to have all or most of the modern amenities, the barbell should be considered an integral part of the home, as exercise should be considered an integral part of healthy living.

Unless well-accustomed to hauling and lifting, when commencing to use the barbell in the dead-lift exercise, it is best to begin with a weight equal to half the exerciser's body-weight.

If that weight can be lifted five times in succession without undue exertion, certainly without obviously increased breathing, such a weight is a sensible commencing weight.

After a week or two of daily use, viz.: five reps, move up, by degrees, if cautious, until ten reps can be done, easily and without any adverse symptoms whatever.

After another week or two of ten reps, add 5 lb. to each end of the barbell, or if strong and ambitious, perhaps 10 lb. to each end, and go back to the routine of five reps, moving up to ten reps over a period of a few weeks.

This procedure can be carried on as long as the effort fulfils the demands as stated in this chapter.

To lift, make sure the feet are under the barbell, the knees well-bent, the body as erect as possible, the head looking straight ahead, and the back flat, certainly not bowed and bent over the barbell. The actual lifting is first done with the legs. When the legs are straightened the body is moved to the fully erect position, and the shoulder-blades caused to meet by pulling the shoulders back. The weight is lowered to the ground by reversing the procedure.

On no account submit to the temptation to lift a very heavy weight until well-conditioned to do so. This may take some years in the case of the man over 40. Even then he is wise to lift within his reasonable limits. Groin, and other strains, can occur.

Never lift after, or within, two hours of a meal. Never lift with a full bladder. Never lift if you have to use your will-power. Lift with your strength but never over-exert. If the slightest palpitation of the heart, or heavy breathing after an effort, whether a single lift, or several reps, the effort is too much for your condition. Go back to lighter weights.

Watch for the slightest sign of groin or lower abdominal strain. Two more 'reps' done on will-power can cause such a strain. Be certain to keep the body as erect as possible and the back flat. Thus the legs do most of the work and are thus strengthened by their isotonic movement. The abdominals and back muscles are also exercised isotonically. The arms are exercised isometrically. In this way *all* the musculative including the neck and shoulders are exercised in some form and beneficially.

Remember, dead-lifting does not really 'exercise' the heart, the heart merely responds to the call made upon it. Therefore, exercise the heart by vigorous walking, running, and some swimming.

Finally, dead-lifting will make you feel fit, well and confident. For this reason alone it is justified, shall we say – a *must*.

Chapter Fourteen

If you grow to love the barbell – here are some more exercises.

I have dealt with the No. 1 exercise – the Dead-lift and sounded the warnings. It is interesting to note that no other heavy lift can cause the risk of strain. It is the Dead-lift that pulls on the long tendons and 'strings' of the abdominals. To a modified extent this can be said of 'cleaning' the barbell.

To 'clean' the exerciser stands over the barbell as in the Dead – lift, but, in one convulsive jerk he moves the barbell off the ground and finds it (hopefully) – resting upon his hands in front of his chest. From this position he can push, or jerk the barbell over his head.

However, both the 'clean and jerk' and 'press' are competitive weight-lifters' movements. Neither of them confer anything worthwhile on the exerciser. For him, as for the competing weight-lifter, these lifts can only be an evidence of strength and technique.

For actual exercising it is far better to have two dumb-bells, although one will do, to load the dumb-bell(s) up to a suitable weight, and proceed as follows:

Lean over the dumb-bell, legs partly bent at the knee, and pull the dumb-bell off the ground and hoisting it to shoulder level. Do five to ten as strength improves, then add a little more weight, and revert to five reps.

CHAPTER FOURTEEN

The other exercise involves hoisting the dumb-bell to the shoulder, then pushing it above the head with the arm fully extended. After five to ten, and with both arms, add more weight, and revert to five reps.

Another good exercise, especially for the pectorals, those slabs of muscle missing from the chest of most men, is the bench or prone press. This exercise can be done prone on a bench, or prone on the floor. (See photo.)

The barbell is pushed away from the chest to arms length. One disadvantage with this exercise is, when the weight is very heavy, it may have to be lifted into the hands of the exerciser.

Another excellent all-over strengthener, the legs, the abdominals, the back, shoulders and arms, is the Swing. A dumb-bell is used loaded, in the beginning to one fourth, or one-third, of the body-weight. It should be swung five times with each hand, working up to ten reps, as in all other exercises.

When able to handle a heavier weight, do so. There is no risk of strain. In doing this exercise the dumb-bell rests on the floor beneath the body and between the feet. It is lifted clear of the ground so that it can be swung backwards and forwards between the legs. Then, with a strong effort, *keeping the swinging arm straight*, the dumb-bell is swung high over the head to return to the position between the legs.

This exercise is a variation of the Sit-up and Dead-lift exercises, and makes for more fluidity, even though less actual weight is moved.

Perhaps the best single exercise other than the dead-lift could be the 'curl'. The curl, which can be done in what is called the military style, or the cheat style, can be done with the barbell as a two-handed exercise, or with the dumb-bell as an alternate arm single-handed exercise.

The weight, whether barbell or dumb-bell, is held suspended from the straightened arm. With a sudden convulsive jerk the barbell, or the dumb-bell, is swung upwards until the weight is resting level with the upper chest.

This exercise is excellent for the forearm controlling the grip, or handshake muscles, as well as the biceps. When a reasonable heavy weight is used on the barbell, from half the body-weight to body-weight, the effort throws a considerable tension upon the legs, the abdominals and back muscles. This means that the exercise is isometric for all the muscles other than the arms where the muscles are exercised isotonically.

The Dead-lift, and the swing and curl, are the three exercises *par excellence* to strengthen the back and abdominal and arm muscles. With great strength and the consequent tone of the organs and glands, the male will feel greater confidence in his general approach to life, as well as an ability to demonstrate his sexual virility.

It can be accepted as axiomatic that when the male over 40, and possibly when younger, realises the decline of his sexual ability and potency, he will normally attempt to compensate for this by an excess of activity in his business, perhaps, in addition, an over-emphasis on his sport (e.g., golf and fishing), or an unwonted enthusiasm for his social 'do good' or politico-interest activities.

These activities will take him away from his home and his spouse more and more. With a high level of physical strength derived from the exercises suggested, the male, even if he finds his interest in other than connuptial activities increasing, he will be spared the defeatist, inferiority, or compensatory attitudes associated with non-fitness

At worst he will know that what he does is because of choice, rather than an escape that offers no alternative.

This feeling of capacity and strength will strengthen such a man's capacities in his social and business activities. Knowing himself to be a physically strong male he will find a marked lessening of his fears. He will tend to be positive and assertive in his attitudes rather than purely dogmatic: of strong opinions, and less given to compromise and temporising.

He may not find he is making more money, nor perhaps advancing his interests whatever they may be, but he will find he is more content, at least in the recognition that money and status are not the be-all and end-all of living.

But he will find that certain other males, similarly strong, self-reliant, fearless, recognise him and accord him a respect that is not accorded to many other men no matter how academic, wealthy, or otherwise successful.

More gratifying, even if not satisfying, will be the knowledge that he is again, interesting to interesting women, not so much for what he represents, or stands in front of, but what he *is*. It is a proposition that I never doubt that the man who has strengthened his arms with thousands of curls, will, through the strength he enjoys in his arms, especially in the forearm and grip, find himself quite capable of holding his own against all comers, irrespective of size.

It is not suggested that in a civilized society any man need approach life as if he was a powerful ape, but I do say, and definitely, that the only *true* confidence any man can feel arises from his muscle cells.

Confidence, when a man is sick or unfit, is based in his ability to 'buy' strength, or power. Such a man must feel fearful of what will happen to him as a male should he lose his wealth, influence, or power.

The physically strong, that is 'barbell' strong, will never entirely have such fears: such a man realises that, if life reverts to the primitive, as it does in war, and that his form of society and his bulwarks disappear, as they have for the citizens of perhaps one-half of the people living on the globe, he will survive, be able to wrest a livelihood and still be attractive to women.

These attitudes and feelings are deeply seated in the consciousness of all men. For countless thousands of years it was only strong (physically) and fearless men who dominated their fellows. It is the 'peck' theory over again, this time in our human relations.

The recent advent, in the last century or two, of extremely rich men and powerful corporations, the executives of which frequently die before reaching 60 years of age, often in the forties, is no refutation of my statements.

Deprived of their wealth and power such men are deprived of everything they rely upon. It is not to be wondered that such individuals will exploit every possible means, even to the risk of an atomic war. They well might not only destroy themselves, and all their material assets, including cities and the devastation of much of the Earth's surface, but destroy the women and the children, and, naturally, or is it unnaturally, all those males who may be fit, healthy, and not a direct party to such insane attitudes and activities. The very insanity of the possibilities is evidence surely of the fear and the absence of belief in the capacity of all such to cope, physically, since few, or any of them could be considered fit enough to physically protect either their wealth or their positions.

Indeed, in this regard, it is interesting to observe that in two countries involved deeply in certain commitments even the youth called up for national service fail to the order of some 50 per cent to meet the necessary fitness levels for the armed services.

For all thoughtful people this incidence of unfitness is most disconcerting, both to intelligent citizens, as it is to the Governments of Countries.

To me, there is only one solution for the intelligent individual, and that is, to achieve, and retain a fitness that at least supports an attitude of mind that resists the trend to self-destruction since atomic war implies self-destruction as well as destruction of the 'enemy'.

There is a theory, and not without credence, that with the birth of the life-force in an embryo, is born the death force. In the first years of growth the life force is in the ascendancy. Then there would appear to be a period when the two forces, life and death, are approximately

CHAPTER FOURTEEN

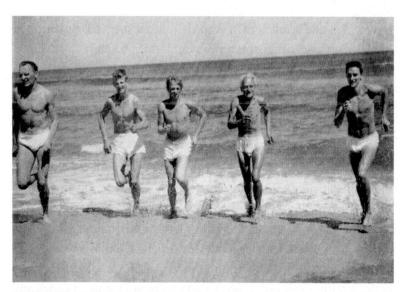

The author leaving the sea with a number of runners – mid-winter

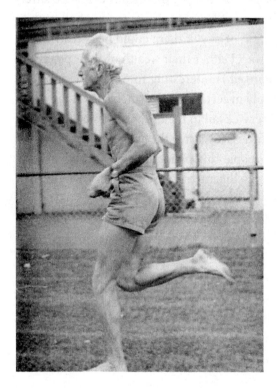

The author running at 70 years of age

CHAPTER FOURTEEN

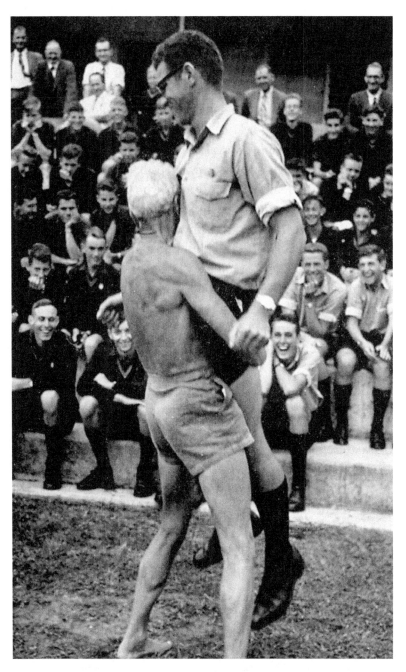

The author, body weight 130 lb (59 kg) lifting a lad weighing 14 stone (196 lb or 89 kg).

CHAPTER FOURTEEN

in balance. This period may last only ten years, 20 years, possibly, at the most, when the forces of dissolution gain the ascendancy. From this point onwards man, as an entity, is on the way out.

That this period of balance can be extended, and the scales stopped from tipping in the direction of dissolution cannot now be doubted. But the balance is only held by maintaining the physical body at a certain level of health and physical fitness. Once that level drops below the safe mean a man is on the downward path to his grave.

It is trite to remark that no man who is in perfect health and balance today, tomorrow suddenly becomes physically and organically decrepit, other than through accident. The heart does not collapse overnight. The condition that ends in a coronary, or a stroke has been developing for years. Kidneys and livers, like abdominals and biceps, do not become weak and ineffective, unable to cope, in a week or a year.

Indeed, there are indications, levels, and measurements which can be a reliable guide. These will be dealt with.

Summary of Chapter Fourteen

Extra exercises, using the barbell, and the dumb-bell, are:
1. The 'clean': a barbell is violently pulled upwards off the ground to a position where it rests upon the hands close to the upper chest and under the chin. This exercise can be repeated, or
2. Be completed with the 'Jerk', when the barbell is jerked overhead with an upward thrust of the arms whilst at the same time the body dips downwards to help the movement. The legs can remain together or split.
   The Clean and Jerk, which is one of the three competitive exercises, can be done one handed with a dumb-bell, and this may indeed be preferable as a pure exercise.

3. Dumb-bell 'Pumps'. A dumb-bell is placed on the ground, seized with one hand, and pulled upwards to shoulder height. It is different to the Clean as the body remains bent over and the wrists do not cock over.
4. ' Prone or Bench Presses': executed on a bench or upon the floor. The exerciser lies prone and pushes the weight away from the chest.
5. The 'Swing' ; a dumb-bell is placed between the feet upon the ground, grasped, lifted clear of the ground and swung first of all backwards and forwards once or twice to gain impetus, and then, with the arm held straight, the dumb-bell is swung over the head.
6. The 'Curl', done with the 'chest', or free-movement technique. A barbell, or dumb-bell is held suspended from the arm(s), and in a convulsive movement, in which the body moves freely, the weight is lifted to chest level.

These exercises will provide all that is reasonably required for this form of exercising. Practically all the muscles of the whole organism are exercised either isometrically or isotonically.

The proposition is that the organs and glands tend to take their tone from the well-exercised and powerful muscles contiguous to them, and that, basically, confidence arises from the muscle cells and is felt in the mind, rather than being found through mind action itself. Where there is little physical health, well-being and muscular strength there must be deep fears.

Where there are deep fears, and security and life itself felt to depend upon wealth and power, the mind will evince, in times of stress, panic and desperation. These emotional states can be the cause that results in atomic warfare and the destruction of much of the earth and its peoples.

A further proposition is that in the period of growth, from the embryo to adulthood, the life-force in us can be said to be in the ascendancy with the death-force that is also born with us. After a period, varying considerably with different individuals, and dependent, this writer believes, upon the degree of physical fitness, muscularity and organ health, the two forces are in balance.

But this period of balance passes and the death-force, bringing about ultimate dissolution, gains the ascendancy. From then on there is a slow, or rapid, deterioration of organ function ending in eventual dissolution.

That this process can be slowed up, even arrested, and lost ground recovered, is beyond question or doubt. Indeed, the degree to which this process of dissolution can be retarded has not yet been fully tested. But there is no doubt that an organism fed upon suitable aliment, and efficiently exercised, can be expected to, perhaps, double the span usually expected in our form of civilization. It can be taken as axiomatic that – 'Only the Fit are Fearless': that 'Healthy organs and powerful muscles fight for us better than guns and bombs': that 'where there is genuine physical fitness, in that country, and that individual, "reason", not power, will be King'.

Definitely, and finally – 'Fitness Pays'.

Chapter Fifteen

Some measure-rods: criteria and means of determining the degree of fitness, together with the indications and warnings that precede unfitness and early or eventual demise short of what might have been.

If you are a fit man, muscularly and organically, when you are sitting at your office· table, or in other ways inactive, and have been inactive, perhaps, for one hour, you may take your pulse.

This is easily done with a stop-watch, or a watch or other time-piece with a second, or sweep hand. If, after several such tests, you average 70 pulse beats per minute, you can believe you are reasonably, even normally, fit.

If you record a pulse rate in the low sixties you are exceptionally fit, need have no worry as to heart attacks (other factors being equal as they almost certainly will be), and can expect to enjoy any reasonable physical activity open to you. This means, any form of sport, mountain-walking, swimming, and competitively in sport if you have aspirations, and irrespective of age.

If you take your basic or basal pulse rate, as it is termed, and this is done on awaking after a night's rest, and before even sitting up (so you need to have your stop-watch or other means of timing handy), and you record your pulse rate in the low fifties, again, you will know you are very fit, and well able to extend

CHAPTER FIFTEEN

yourself competitively in any sport, e.g., tennis, football, cricket, table-tennis, competitive walking or running races, if you are so inclined.

If you take your basic pulse rate (as above) and you find the rate is in the low forties per minute, you are fit to compete as athletically as you have the strength and technique to do so, whether it is competitive rowing, mile or marathon racing, or competing at Wimbledon in tennis! Unless, of course, there is some definite slowing up of the pulse rate due to weakness, and you are about to die!

If you are above 70 beats per minute whilst resting, you are well-advised to do something about it. It is true, you may not die before 80 or 90 years of age because you are over 70 beats at 40 years of age, but, frankly, I would not like your chances.

Moreover, without a powerful slow-beating heart, even if you live, you will not be one of the vital, active type, therefore, missing, surely, the physical enjoyment that could be open to you. There is virtue in being able to enjoy a 'game with the kids': to play your part in a world that was, and still is, physical, and long before the development of the brain.

If you find your movements have slowed up: or you puff and pant with the slightest unusual hurrying or activity, you are on the way out: in the vernacular, the skids are under you. On the other hand it is normal to breathe deeply with any extra exertion. Even a short burst of 50 yards will cause heavier breathing, but any effort, whether 50 yards, three hundred, or three miles, that causes faintness, dizziness or nausea, suggests you are not fit for the effort. The first two are bad signs. The last is not unusual when the effort is to the point of exhaustion. Therefore, it is commonplace for athletes and others to feel a nausea, or sick feeling in the stomach, if the exertion has been extreme and to the point of exhaustion. However, there still should be no dizziness or faintness.

There is no special advantage in being able to touch your toes, or put your palms on the floor. All that indicates is that your joints, and it applies to all joints, since they will all follow the same pattern – all your joints lock late. With some people their joints lock early. They can never really straighten their extended arm, or leg, and when they bend over, find it difficult, if not impossible to touch their toes.

It is true, constant stretching, and constant bending, will keep the joints fully responding, but like being double-jointed, there is no special benefit to be derived, other than, perhaps, being a gymnast or a contortionist. It is true, unless we bend and exercise, the muscles and joints can tighten up until, in old age, it may be difficult to bend sufficiently to tie one's shoe-lace.

All muscular exercise constricts, or shortens, the muscles used. It is necessary to counter this as one ages, to stretch all limbs, and the trunk, as does a cat, after resting. The most efficient, for humans, is to hang from a horizontal bar. The hands grip the bar, but every other muscle is relaxed and the body draws out and sinks to the ground by gravity. It is not unusual to find that, over a time period of one minute, the body will so stretch that the feet have moved two, three, or four inches nearer to the ground, as the body lengthens.

Extreme physical effort, such as running at full pace up a hill, or any other exercise, approximating the same severity, can cause a movement of the bowels. Indeed, any vigorous exercise can cause the same reaction, especially running early in the morning. Probably, this is as good a relief from constipation as any other.

Vigorous exercise will cause a certain amount of discomfort, soreness, even stiffness, in the muscles involved. Curiously enough, another dose of the cause undertaken at a lesser tempo, is the best 'cure' for such soreness, or stiffness. Again, however, if the case is severe, it may be necessary to rest the affected muscle for a day or two until the extreme soreness abates. This can be determined by trial and error. It is always best to try active movement before rest is resorted to.

If the heart is strong, and the blood-pressure normal, no exercise can be undertaken that can strain the heart, since a healthy

CHAPTER FIFTEEN

heart has an overload capacity half as great again as any load that the heart can be submitted to. If the loads are too heavy, strains, sprains, even ruptures will be experienced long before the heart is seriously, much less permanently damaged. Nevertheless, the wise man over 30 years of age, will have a medical check-up every year or two, since such check-ups are a far more sensible insurance than life assurance policies. Bar a fatal accident the fit man who has reached 90 years or one hundred is most unlikely to need, or his descendants, what has accrued from a life-policy only paid at death. Policies that mature at 40, 50, 60 or 70 years may be quite a different matter, a wise provision and an advantageous increment.

It is now known that muscles that are regularly exercised remain in good tone, and efficient, far longer than muscles that are little exercised, or not used vigorously at all. The story of the talents is true as to muscles and fitness, and their result – longevity. Buried talents, that is unexercised muscles, even if not defective, gain no increment. Only the muscles, like capital, that are put to work, gain, grow, or return a dividend.

Evidence of above usual fitness will be demonstrated, unless tired, or depressed mentally, by quick movements, vigorous activity when necessary, and an instinctive desire to 'do' things, e.g., go for a brisk walk : a run : to skate: to ski: swim : play games. All such motivations can be deemed normal and natural, and to an advanced age.

Such impulses should not be resisted. If possible, a part of the programme for each day should be so channelled. When all is said and done, 'Life is Movement', and 'Variety of Movement is the Spice of it'.

Summary of Chapter Fifteen

You will know you are physically fit heart-wise if, when resting, e.g., sitting at a desk, and after so minutes or so resting, your pulse rate is not more than 70 beats per minute.

CHAPTER FIFTEEN

If the P.R. is down, in the low sixties, and you are not about to die, that is, your P.R. is low because you are so weak, in any case you would be so weak you would probably be in bed, then you can view yourself as an unusually fit man, whatever your age, and almost any exercise or work your muscles can do for you, you are free to attempt it.

A proviso is that you are found to have a normal blood pressure, certainly, in the Systolic or upper reading, a plus or minus no greater than ten above the normal, at any age, and which is – 120.

Your Basic Pulse Rate, or B.P.R., and which is taken upon waking, but before rising, is the true indication of your strength-stamina factor. If it is in the low forties, you are capable of submitting your organism (body and muscles) to almost any effort, in any sport, muscle strains or sprains excepted.

If in the low fifties, you are still fitter than most young people and can haul, hike, run or climb mountains with most, young or old.

If in the low sixties, your B.P.R. indicates you are in normal health and fitness but very hard exertions should not be undertaken, at least, precipitately. If your B.P.R is only 70 or over, after you have lain prone for several hours, although you may not drop dead on rising, you are little likely to be able to enjoy, without symptoms of faintness, or distress, any extreme exertion.

A high blood pressure, e.g., 130/140 systolic, is getting on the dangerous side. You may feel well, most H.B.P. people do – but they often drop dead, or have a stroke. Your job is to get your B.P.R. and B.P. down to normal, or healthy, limits. Do not take any notice of the highly dangerous statement that your B.P. is okay if it is said to be one hundred plus your age. I think it is a perfectly safe statement you will never find a man 90 years of age with a B.P. of 190, nor one with a B.P. of 200 at 100 years of age. People with such B.P's have died long before those ages.

In any case, with a high P.R. and a high B.P. such a person, when aged, does not 'live': they merely are still with us. Surely, there is a distinction to be made here.

CHAPTER FIFTEEN

Faintness: Dizziness: infusion of blood to the face and neck: or extreme bleaching of the face – these are the chief warning signs, as are panting, puffing, coughing, staggering or collapsing. Never reach these stages in an over-exuberance or foolish enthusiasm. Set about becoming physically fit, when such states are almost impossible to reach.

Palpitations of the heart in the chest are perhaps the warning of warnings, as can be a heavy pulse on the temple. When the heart is powerful it is never felt unless the hand is placed over it when it may be felt pounding, otherwise, there is no evidence at all that it is being worked, or exerted, even to its maximum effort.

Make stretching all your limbs part of your routine. Sitting on the floor one can stretch out to reach each spread foot, or stretch and bend over to touch toes, but the best stretching is done hanging by the grip from a horizontal bar and letting gravity, NOT muscular effort, pull you out.

A piece of pipe, three feet long and two inches in diameter, can often be easily and readily fixed all to a wall, or other upright, and is invaluable as part of the 'Home Gym'. It is useful for doing 'Chins' also, when by exerting the arms the chin is lifted to bar level.

Stiffness and soreness of exercised muscles is customary and not serious. When not too bad, the 'cure' is in more of the exercise that caused the soreness.

Get a medical check-up every other year or so, especially as to the heart and blood pressure.

Move fast: Be brisk: respond to the instinct to exercise, whether it be to walk, run, swim, climb. Remember 'LIFE IS MOVEMENT'. (Nothing else.)

Chapter Sixteen

A daily exercise schedule for the busy man prepared to devote no more than 15 minutes per day to his fitness. In the beginning we must assume his weight is reasonably normal, and his heart passed by his doctor.

To start his day he should, on rising, before or after his daily shave and shower (*before* could be better), lie down on the floor, place his feet under a piece of furniture, or something similar that will keep his feet down, and do his daily sit-ups.

He should be able to do five sit-ups as a minimum, ten is better. If he wants to exceed ten, he can only benefit by so doing up to any number – 100 or more – just as long as there are no feelings of exhaustion, infusion of blood to the face and neck, or other than a deep breathing rhythm, i.e., no panting.

The first thing to do when prone on the floor is to fully fill the lungs. Then, as the body is lifted to the sitting position the air in the lungs is exhaled. The body is forced towards the now drawn-up knees by pressure from the hands on the back of the head. Every effort being made to force all the air from the lungs, deliberately and consciously. Two or three forward jerks can be done to emphasize this complete emptying of the lungs.

As the body returns to the prone position and the pressure is thus removed from the abdomen and the lower chest area, so will the lungs fill with air again.

This exercise, when it becomes normal and habitual, will ensure that the lungs are reasonably cleansed of residual air, and will start up a deeper breathing rhythm that should be maintained throughout the day.

Also, the heart will return to a higher rate of pulse ready for the day's work and the efforts, even if only of walking, and which is essential after the lowered pulse rate whilst in bed sleeping.

Thus the heart and circulatory system are made ready for the day and a deeper breathing rhythm started up. It is interesting to note here that an early morning cigarette can be expected to have exactly the same effect, viz. : an increased heart beat and pulse rate, and a quickened breathing rate, the deeper rhythm being usually incited in order to clear the accumulated mucous from the throat and bronchial passages. But just how harmful this can be to both the heart and the lungs only the increasing incidence of heart disease and cancer of the lungs can statistically prove.

The increased breathing rhythm and the higher pulse rate, both due to the exercise will make for an increased wakefulness and energy, a feeling of well-being and an optimism as to the day's tasks.

It is to be noted that because of their high blood pressure and higher pulse rates that hypertension sufferers usually feel quite energetic and optimistic on rising. These are the people who bustle around, seem to be always busy, or in a hurry, and evince above ordinary optimism and drive.

However, these very conditions are a warning rather than an advantageous condition, and should be so considered, when there is a blood pressure above 140 m.g., certainly above 150.

It is far better, because the pulse rate is low and the blood-pressure normal, to awake feeling lethargic, since very little movement, certainly a few minutes exercise, will bring both the pulse rate and the blood-pressure up to levels making for an efficient day's work, and well within the capacity of the heart to handle all reasonable requirements, no matter what other muscles may tire or become stiff and sore through being over-exercised.

Therefore, some exercise, whether it be five or ten, or so, sit-ups, a short run, a brisk walk, or a few minutes skipping – all or any will be advantageous on rising:[1]

Allow 3 minutes

Time left 12 minutes

Assuming a sedentary job, if the person is fit, it will be normal and natural to seize every opportunity to enjoy a little more exercise during the day. This can take the form of quick walks to various parts of the office, or works, rather than communicating per the house telephone system, or summoning another to one's desk or office. Use the stairs rather than the lift. It should not be difficult to achieve another three minutes of fairly vigorous exercise in this manner, so we can allow another

3 minutes

Time left 9 minutes

However, the major part of the day that can be availed of brisk walking would be the lunch period. It should be possible, most days, no matter what the arrangements may be, what the calls or appointments, to arrange to walk vigorously for half-a-mile, or thereabouts. Such a burst of vigorous exercise, taken in the middle of the day, and before consuming a light salad and protein

---

[1] It cannot be sufficiently emphasized that, whilst an increasingly high systolic blood-pressure reading would appear to be the normal expectancy, the author definitely states that this need not be so: that such a condition as hypertension is abnormal, and because hypertension victims so often show recordings as high as 180, even over 200, it is entirely erroneous to assume any normality in the old acceptance of 100 plus one's age. Persons who accord with such readings at 60 years of age are little likely to survive to record 180 at 80 years, and certainly – *never* 200 at 100 years of age.

CHAPTER SIXTEEN

lunch, can be expected to stimulate the heart's action and set the pace for the rest of the day's work.

For the midday exercise

Allow 6 minutes
Time left 3 minutes

The three minutes still remaining could be best utilised by a short brisk walk, a jog of even as short a distance as 200 yards, or metres, or three minutes of skipping, or a few sit-ups immediately before going to bed.

Allow 3 minutes
Time exhausted

If a day's exercise, or part of the day's 15 minutes is missed for any reason, the lost exercise time should be added to the following day's programme. The essential thing is to make sure a weekly total of at least 1 ½ hours *vigorous* exercise is taken each week, and spread over as many days as possible.

This regime, whilst it is the simplest possible, should be considered the absolute minimum if any person would remain healthy, fit and active, certainly after 40 years of age, probably after 30 years of age.

Attention to diet should be maintained, and the bodyweight controlled through diet, since the amount of exercise suggested will have little or no effect in reducing weight, indeed, the healthy feeling of well-being can be expected to cause a healthy feeling of appetite. But as has been explained there are no problems as to diet if the starches are eliminated, or almost eliminated, .from the diet.[1]

The 15 minutes per day regime can be considered sufficient exercise to enable a person to enjoy occasional long walks of two or three hours duration, or covering in distance five or six miles, even further.

This means a person can be expected to enjoy the exercise

---

1 Vegetables and fruits, even potatoes, need never be considered as 'starches'. Starches refer to bread, biscuits, and all manufactured products using flour or similar as a base. This will include most puddings, cakes, buns and pastries.

CHAPTER SIXTEEN

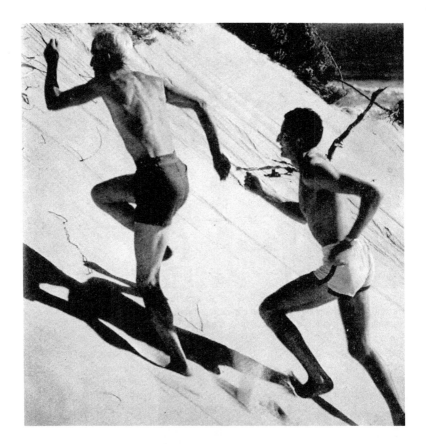

The author running on the sand hill at Portsea with his pupil, Herb Elliott, a world-record breaking athlete.

CHAPTER SIXTEEN

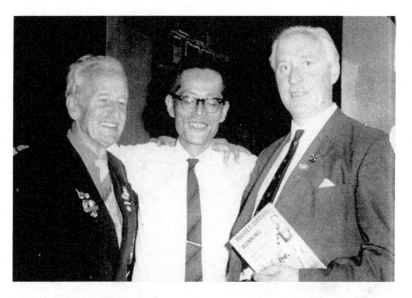

The author with his publisher, William Luscombe, and a newspaper editor in Tokyo, for the Olympic Games 1964

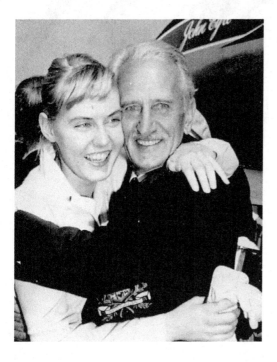

The author with his step-daughter Elaine, taken upon return from Tokyo.

associated with golf, certainly playing bowls, and even tennis could be played to, at least, 60 years of age, all other factors being reasonably satisfied.

These factors are only little or no over-weight, a resting pulse rate of 70 or a little more, and a blood-pressure not higher than 140 systolic.

Basically, what is required to maintain any such regime as to exercise and eating is – SELF DISCIPLINE. The reward for this self-discipline can be considered three-fold.

They are:
1. To ensure above average longevity enjoyed reasonably free from ill health and degenerative diseases.
2. The ability to enjoy weekend sport, gardening or other activities.
3. The enjoyment of a feeling of well-being free of known disease or disability, together with the knowledge that the occasional 'breaking of the rules' is not likely to be 'punished' by a heart attack or similar collapses or seizures.

Summary of Chapter Sixteen

Assume a normal weight, certainly not more than ten pounds over-weight, and your doctor certifies that your heart is O.K., and blood-pressure satisfactory, then-

On rising, programme for five to ten sit-ups (or more) breathing deeply whilst the exercise is being done. Inhale as the body sinks to the floor and exhale as completely as possible as the body rises and is forced between the knees.

This exercise sets up a good heart rhythm and breathing rhythm for the day, as well as exercising the abdominals and back especially.

A brisk walk, a short jog, three minutes skipping, or a cigarette – can be expected to send up the pulse rate also. But the cigarette, being a toxic drug, will shorten your life: the exercises as stated will certainly tend to lengthen your expectation.

Man, like all animals, tends to wake up sleepily, i.e., feeling lethargic. This is because the pulse rate has slowed by resting, and the blood-pressure has fallen. Therefore, this is natural.

It is only the hypertension patient who awakens feeling fit and well, energetic and ready for the day's activity. Actually this is a pathological state. Such people are not to be envied.

The before breakfast exercises need take no more than three minutes, so –

Allow 3 minutes
Minutes remaining 12

At the office, or works, if the occupation is sedentary, take every opportunity to move away from your table or desk, walk briskly and use the stairs rather than the lift.

Allow 3 minutes
Minutes remaining 9

The lunch interval is the chance to walk briskly, deliberately breathing deeply, thus regenerating the system for the afternoon's work.

Allow 6 minutes
Minutes remaining 3

The balance of time, vig. 3 minutes can be used in a short run, a skip, or some sit-ups, before returning.

Extra years expected from some such regime – *five to ten* at the very minimum over an otherwise reasonable expectancy, and then – *fit* extra years.

All that is required, in addition, is a sitting (resting) pulse rate of around 70: a systolic blood pressure, preferably not above 130, certainly not above 140, little or no overweight – and all that is in Life – can be yours.

Chapter Seventeen

A daily exercise schedule for the man prepared to devote 30 minutes per day to his fitness and physical well-being.

I believe it has been proved that the Heart muscle needs steady and rhythmic exercising. Nothing is more conducive to achieve this end than steady running.

Walking is good but it requires much more time for its performance. The physical benefit to be derived from 30 minutes pleasant running can be equal to two or three hours walking.

Since time is a factor in most transactions few busy men will afford the time to exercise their hearts for as long as 30 minutes each day.

But since we are as 'old', and most things being equal as they are, we live as long as our hearts continue to beat – exercising the heart regularly (and protecting it from toxins), is a far better insurance for life than buying it.

I then suggest, for the 'vigorous exercise man' who is prepared to devote 30 minutes per day to his fitness, that he will regularly do his sit-up exercise, as will the 15 minute day schedule man, but will add five minutes of vigorous skipping, or even better, a run involving the same time, viz., five minutes.

These two exercises alone can be expected to keep the waistline trim (the diet, of course, being reasonable and controlled) and the heart in first-class condition for all normal purposes.

CHAPTER SEVENTEEN

The pulse rate will be brought up to a normal rate, viz., between 60 and 70 beats per minute – when sitting, and the blood-pressure within the stated limits, viz. under 140 m.g. systolic, preferably under 130.

Naturally, for such a man, willing to exercise in this manner and for the time required – Nicotine (smoking) will be completely banned. Otherwise the load placed on the Nicotine affected heart can, sooner or later, create a condition that might easily have a serious result.

It cannot be emphasized sufficiently that the older man who would exercise hard: who would be active and fit, as he well might be – and far above the usually observed level, and who would enhance his life expectancy – he cannot expect to safely embark upon such an exercise schedule, and to continue the schedule into old age, that is – over 60 or 70 years of age – and continue to poison his blood stream, his whole organic system, as well as his heart – by the use of Nicotine in any form, or any quantity.

Stated in axiomatic form, but subject to a reasonable dietary and alcohol intake: Exercise preserves life: Nicotine kills. Or in other words – Exercise *extends* one's life expectancy: Nicotine, definitely and positively *shortens* the life expectancy.

Having performed his sit-ups, and in other ways, such as a five minute run or skip – the Exerciser finds he has exhausted some ten minutes of his scheduled 30 minutes.

         Time used 10 minutes
         Time remaining 20 minutes

At his office or works (we assume as most function – a sedentary occupation), he will take every opportunity to move from point to point, and his usual movement from floor to floor being via the stairs, and hopefully ascended – two at a time.[1]

---

[1] The author in his seventy second year is still able to run a stairway of 116 stairs, each of a seven inch rise, and equivalent to a six-storey building, two steps at a time without any strain upon his heart, and nothing more than heavy breathing when the run is completed. The run is not done slowly or laboriously, but as fast as possible.

CHAPTER SEVENTEEN

The exerciser can expect to get at least five minutes brisk exercise in this manner. This means the time allotted exercising is reduced by – 5 minutes

Time remaining 15 minutes

Such a programme leaves 15 minutes, each day. Another five minutes can be utilised with a brisk walk at luncheon time, but it is far better to consider any such activity as outside the programme and to devote the remaining time, viz. 15 minutes, to much more strenuous exercising. This could take the form, one day, of 15 minutes, devoted to lifting heavy weights, i.e. barbell work, or a mile or two running on the other day.

The barbell work could be:

5 to 10 'Reps' in the Dead-lift with 100 lb.

5 to 10 'Reps' using each arm – of the one-handed swing

5 to 10 'Curls' using the 'free' movements.

Use a weight that makes the exercise possible but not easy

(N.B.: Re-read Chapters 13 and 14.)

It becomes important if a person is to fulfil this programme that he commences his jogging as soon as possible, and when he is able to – to move to the order of continuous running, even if done slowly, for 15 minutes.

For any man over 40 years of age – two miles run in 15 minutes can be considered first-class as to fitness and warrants an 'A' certificate.

Such a programme of exercise reasonably pursued from 30 years of age to 50 years of age, and subject always to keeping the weight to a fitness level and no Nicotine toxins, can mean that the man without any congenital or incipient disease can be expected to play any sport, no matter how hard or active, and at first-class levels.

If, after 50 or 60 years of age, the programme is modified to half the weekly output and the same attention paid to the dietary habits, then the fitness level required for a continuation of squash, tennis, golf or similar sports can be expected to be enjoyed until well into the seventies and eighties.

This prognostication must be, as it will be, subject to inherited congenital weakness. But even where the family history is one of poor survival expectancy, experience has shown that the historical factor in all ordinary cases can be completely ignored; that each individual creates his own destiny and determines his longevity much more than was believed in medical circles only as short a time ago as 20 years.

With the development and acceptance of the evolutionary theory as first propounded by Darwin last century, it was natural that much more emphasis .was placed on the hereditary factor than is now accepted.

Actually, for all normal creatures, it is the environmental factor that is by far the most important. Fed wrongly, especially on factorised foods or unsuitable foods, a baby born with an hereditary expectancy of 70 or 80 years may find it is dead in one year.[1]

Or an adult with a similar expectancy because of the longevity of parents and grandparents may find that a 'heart' condition has intervened as early as in the forties.

All such instances can be attributed to the environmental factors, not the hereditary factor. Finally, it can be stated that the man who has bothered to maintain his physical organism on the lines suggested, until he dies – whether that be under or over one hundred years – will be active enough to care for himself, even do a reasonable amount of laborious work, enjoy some moderate sport, and as is known in countries such as Hunza – procreate his species.

It is also known, and proved, that when the fitness is

---

[1] It is becoming known that babies reared on artificial foods from birth are going to exhibit heart and artery conditions to an unfavourable degree as compared with babies wholly, or partly, breast fed. This could be said of mothers who smoke and who take drugs when pregnant, or lactating.

CHAPTER SEVENTEEN

maintained by some attention to exercise – even if not programmed, or regular, the ability to do heavy exercise, e.g., running (not jogging or ambling) but running a mile under eight minutes, or five, perhaps, in 40 minutes, climbing hills without undue breathlessness, and lifting his body-weight in repetitions, as well as swimming, surfing, and much else, can be normal for a septuagenarian.[1]

Summed up, and in conclusion, the scientific and medical world up to the present time, has been so preoccupied with the things of the world that the things of the spirit, meaning the Life Principle in us, has almost entirely been neglected.

The medical profession, preoccupied as it has been with sickness, and disease – in a word, keeping mankind free of contagious diseases and induced sicknesses, has left the matter of physical fitness almost entirely to a few enthusiasts, popularly termed 'fitness cranks'.

Nevertheless, these fitness enthusiasts are proving to be the pathfinders into the field of geriatrics, that branch of medicine concerned with the aged. It can be said with certainty that when medicine has finished its task, if ever, on the problems of world-wide malnutrition, induced diseases, such as coronaries and cancers, and turns its attention in sufficient numbers and time to the subject of health and fitness in middle and old-age, the life expectancy as now experienced may well be doubled.

But the wise man will not wait for this medical miracle to happen. He will realise his potentiality: the possibilities: and carve his own road to a healthy, fit and useful agedness through – .

Controlled food intake: elimination of harmful and toxic substances and some programmed exercise done as a self-imposed duty – and for its own sake.

---

[1] The author demonstrates these evidences of fitness without any regular daily programme, or any programme for that matter.

CHAPTER SEVENTEEN

Summary of Chapter Seventeen

The heart muscle, it is known, requires regular exercising. Running is the exercise *par excellence.*

Walking is time consuming: three hours walking can be considered equivalent to 30 minutes running.

Actually a man is as 'old' as his heart and arteries. If his heart and arteries are maintained in good health and condition he remains 'young' – even at 70 years of age.

Nicotine can be considered the main 'killer', since it affects the heart, the next is over-eating.

For a man willing to commit himself to 30 minutes a day programmed exercise it is suggested:

5-10 sit-ups on rising.

5 minutes skipping, or running.

At office, or works, brisk walking and stair running.

Lunch-hour brisk walking and breathing.

Later in the day –

15 minutes heavy weight-work with barbell or-

15 minutes running.

For extra measure – 5 – 10 sit-ups before retiring.

Such a programme reasonably pursued from 30 to 50 years of age, controlling the appetite especially as to starch foods, and the alcohol intake, can mean a degree of fitness that makes participation in all or any sport possible.

It will also ensure a degree of fitness at 60 and 70 years not usually deemed possible.

If you have a bad family history of sickness or longevity – forget it. If not deeply involved by congenital defects, both your level of fitness and longevity, are reasonably much more under your control than has been previously realised.

Agedness can be kept back, and to a remarkable degree. At 30 years of age you may not think these matters are important.

CHAPTER SEVENTEEN

Before 50, with a 'heart', a coronary, or a cancer it may be too late to recover the lost ground.

Why not swim, lift weights, play squash and tennis, walk up mountains, at 70? Life can be good at 70, even better at 80, for the fit and virile.

Do not rely on the medical profession. Concerned with sickness and disease the profession has not had time to study and prescribe physical fitness and the means of attaining it.

The prescription is simple: A controlled appetite (little or no starches in pure form). No intake of harmful and toxic materials or drugs, of which Nicotine is the most deadly in common usage.

Some fairly regular programmed exercise enjoyed for its own sake, and the vitality that can follow.

Chapter Eighteen

On Ageing.

As we age a balance has to be arrived at between wearing out and rusting out. A marked unbalance in one or the other direction will definitely shorten the expectancy of life for each person.

Too often it is said that 'work never kills'. Overwork carries with it destructive elements. Each person has to achieve his own balance since the amount of energy available for expenditure, the amount of exercise that can be healthily tolerated, and the maximum amount of exercise that provides the optimum fitness, will vary from individual to individual, no two persons being exactly alike.

Therefore, it is wrong to base our needs, or our capacities, upon the needs and capacities of another. As in foods, so in exercise, one man's satisfactory efforts can prove disastrous to another.

Fortunately, there are signs and evidences as to what is reasonably satisfactory. If you are living a reasonably exercised life, your weight will remain steady from day to day, month to month and year to year. There should be no increase at all each year, or decade.

The fit weight will tend to remain stable until 70 years or 80 years of age when, with a declining physical output; the bulk of the muscles can be expected to diminish. Thus, over 70 or 80 years of age, there will be a slight decline in weight, probably not more than 1 lb. per year, but nevertheless, a slight decline.

This could mean that an active, fit man of 70 or 80, and who may have a fit, lean body-weight of 150 lb. could find his body-weight has fallen to 140 lb. at 80 or 90 years of age. This body-weight could remain fairly stable for the next decade or so, when, as the life forces run down, the natural loss of appetite and abandonment of exercise, could cause another fall in body-weight to, perhaps, as low as 130 lb.

However, these falls in weight will be arrested just as much as the person exercises and leads a normally useful life.

There is no evidence to prove that, given a good longevity inheritance, the environmental factors favourable, aliment understood and controlled, a continuing interest in living, and a daily modicum of exercise, the weight norm may be carried over the 100 years and the life expectancy increased to, at least, 120 years.

When the factors for longevity are being reasonably satisfied another evidence will be that persons who meet us for the first time will place our age lower than it is, and comment on our 'youngness' and, absence of the usual evidences of age, viz., slowness of movements, stiffness in the joints, lacklustre, or bloodshot eyes, wrinkled, colourless, or dry facial skin, pendulous flesh on the upper body and abdomen, unnaturally white, bloodless lower limbs, or varicose veins, or blue-veined marbling of the limbs.

Add lifeless hair, if any, and excessive growth of hair in ears and nostrils, together with a secondary eyebrow growth, and we have all the evidences of agedness, that can, at least, be arrested.

Another evidence of the holding back of age will be seen in a genuine interest in those factors that constitute life, and living it. These factors are: ambition, desire for mental and educational improvement, plans for work, especially creative work, an increasing disinterest in time-wasting pursuits, such as sporting activities, e.g., golf and bowls, although these can be a factor in advancing longevity in some, and above all, keeping alive the desire to travel and experience.

Fast reactions and quick movements, especially walking as fast, or faster at the normal city pavement pace, except perhaps, when over-tired, is another certain evidence of aged-fitness.

Above all, there will be little or no evidence, no matter how advanced the age, of senility, brain deterioration, or noticeable decline of the faculties. The pulse rate will be good, hopefully not above 70 beats per minute when resting, and the blood-pressure little above the normal expectancy of 80-120.

Above all, and finally, the person who has arrested agedness will 'feel' young: will 'act' young, but not necessarily juvenile, although there will be a capacity for fun, on occasion: and will feel shocked when, upon looking at themselves in the mirror, they realise that their physiognomy betrays their heart, attitudes, and feelings.

In a word, they may 'look' old, but their 'heart' will be young, their body active, and their brain keen and alert.

Summary of Chapter Eighteen

Age requires a balance between wearing out and rusting out. Either, in excess, shortens life. The essential 'balance' varies with each individual. Discover for yourself your balance. Do not slavishly copy others.

A steady weight factor is usually an evidence of fitness, but after 70 or 80 years it is normal for a slight decline in weight to be evidenced.

However, given all the factors that make for longevity, there is no reason why a steady fit weight, and reasonable activity, cannot be maintained until 100 years and over. For longevity, as well as the body being physically fit, the brain must be active, and the mind still bent on ambition, increased knowledge, and directed to the future. Senility, like general deterioration, can be postponed almost indefinitely, probably indefinitely, in some cases.

Those who have arrested the onslaught of agedness will not only 'feel' young, but will 'look' much younger than their actual years.

There is no better survival factor than a young heart, a lower than normal pulse rate and blood pressure, a keen mind, and a genuine interest in the world around us.

Chapter Nineteen

Human elimination.

Many human ills, certainly when the food intake is reasonably satisfactory, are due to faulty elimination.

It can be truly said that 'perfect' elimination is as important as 'perfect' food intake.

Good, or to express it better, 'perfect' elimination, is dependent upon several conditions. This essential condition should offer no problems to the readers of this book who adopt the simple, but imperative, suggestions therein.

Thus for perfect daily elimination it can be proposed:

1. The intake of ample fluids. The intake will depend upon climate, exercise, and perhaps a natural tendency to sweat. A minimum under normal conditions as to climate and exercise can be considered one and a half pints to two quarts of fluid per day.

If the intake is not sufficient to maintain the body's needs, the normal fluidity of the bowel excrement will suffer, the needed fluid being reabsorbed, and the stools becoming hard and dry.

A too long periodicity, the normal passage through the alimentary canal from mouth to anus being, in general, 24 hours, if this periodicity is exceeded the same trouble may be experienced as occurs with a deficient fluid intake.

Too much is made of the bodily system becoming 'Waterlogged' if the intake of fluid is too great, but in healthy conditions there is no fear of this state, dropsical or otherwise, since the body has the means of getting rid of all reasonable excess via the kidneys and bladder.

It is too commonly believed that one visit to the toilet, or stool elimination, is normal and sufficient. This is not necessarily so. The first movement may, or may not, be a complete elimination of the matter to be excreted. It is more likely, after the lower bowel has been emptied, that a further descent will make a second, even a third visit to the toilet necessary.

It cannot be sufficiently emphasised that complete elimination is a most important factor in maintaining health, removing the possibility of degenerative and other diseases, and ensuring a long, trouble-free maturity into a century-old agedness.

2. To ensure perfect physical functions there must be perfect mental attitudes. The first of these is the acceptance of the concept, or idea, that the normally healthy human body can handle its own effective elimination without any adventitious aids, whether these be cathartics or enemas.

Merely to rise and move the body is usually sufficient to stimulate bowel action, as it is bladder action. However, it is even more certain when a hot drink is taken on waking, or rising, as it is if the body is exercised by vigorous walking or running.

The true and correct attitude of mind, then, is that Nature in us can cause our organs to function as they should if we adopt the right attitude of mind, and 'feed' the body in a reasonable manner.

3. Assuming the factors in '1' and '2' are satisfied, it is still essential that the muscles of the abdomen that bear down upon the intestines, and the peristaltic action of the intestines themselves, be powerful and of good tone. However, reasonable abdominal exercises such as the 'sit-up' take care of this muscular strength and tonic and nothing further is needed

for complete efficient elimination, which should never be looked upon as a task that occurs, or doesn't occur, often at what we deem inopportune moments. Actually elimination must be considered the next in order to efficient aliment, if we would live a life free of disease, debilitations, and especially those diseases of the circulatory system of which cancer must be considered, with the heart, the chief 'killer' of civilised man.

Therefore, although mentioned in '3', it nevertheless requires a paragraph to itself, the inviolate habit that, when Nature 'telegraphs' through the conscious brain the desire to proceed to elimination, no matter what the circumstances, that call is heeded and acceded to. This means that the life-plan must make this possible, and habits formed that offer no obstructions or postponements.

Nothing is more important, and nothing else so looked upon as incidental, as the immediate need for bowel elimination once the need has reached consciousness.

Strict attention to this factor, alone, will be found to mean, at least 20 years of healthy, active life above the normal life expectancy, and it well might prove to be a much higher figure in terms of survival.

Summary of Chapter Nineteen

'Perfect' elimination is as important as a 'perfect' diet.

Good elimination depends primarily on ample fluid intake. The next important factor in good elimination is the mental attitude: the belief that strong abdominal muscles, healthy intestines, and the habit of 'never delaying': that Nature in us can care for elimination just as our heart, given a modicum of daily exercise and good blood as fuel, can care for our circulation .

When the physical body is in good tone, and the mental states good, then merely to rise is often sufficient to cause the bowels to function.

CHAPTER NINETEEN

A hot drink of any kind is the only stimulant to bowel action that ever should be needed. In health, and the factors outlined being satisfied, there is no more need to consider, or think about, much less worry about it – our bowel action than it is to worry about the functioning of the heart, the bladder, or any other natural and normal function.

Chapter Twenty

The large city destroys: the country gives life.

The growing trend towards larger and larger cities with all the destroying factors that are being slowly realised, but which, nevertheless, are very real, as I have attempted to show earlier in this book, suggests that the wise man, interested in his health, fitness and longevity, will try to counter the destroying elements of the overcrowded city. The wise man, by reverting to, at least, some of the ways of living that existed generally before the age of mechanisation, automobiles, electricity, the supermarket, in a word, all the labour-saving devices of modern city life, cut off: as it often is, from the elements, deprived even of fresh, uncontaminated air.

It is to be accepted that the majority of mankind is destined to live and work most of its life under the artificial conditions of the large modern city. However, there is a solution to all problems: a way out of all dilemmas, if we can but find them.

This, then, is to suggest that one solution to the hazards inseparable from living in a large city, is to acquire a section, or area of land in a rural environment. One half to one acre is suggested.

To this rural holding the city dweller will depart at every possible opportunity and most weekends. But it would defeat its purpose should he, even if he has the financial means to have a House Builder, or Contractor, erect the dwelling, and layout the grounds.

CHAPTER TWENTY

The whole idea is that the owner does as much of the work of building and creating as he reasonably can. The whole object is not to provide a country residence, and then move into it, but to provide the situation where the owner finds an outlet in creative work, mostly with his own hands and brains.

In the highly evolved life of business in a large city, where each person is, mostly, merely a cog in a gigantic machine, to maintain a sense of balance and purpose something more is needed.

So: as much of the work as possible is personally done, and in some cases, the whole of the work of construction, laying out, etc., can be done.

As the project develops, and if the area is large enough and suitable, much return to the natural life that man has lived for centuries can be enjoyed by the cultivation of fruit trees and vegetables.

In addition, if it is possible to arrange for feeding, live-stock can be added.

There are vital reasons for this suggestion. Firstly: such activities provide a natural outlet for repressed emotions and the frustrations of city life.

Secondly: the exercise engendered not only is perfectly natural, but through this engenders a feeling of well-being of the mind or spirit.

Thirdly: nothing entirely replaces, whether a person be a city 'worker' with his hands, or a brain worker, working in the country, enjoying the fresh air, and mastering the environment.

To plan for, and enjoy such a project, can mean a renewal of the vital force in an individual to a degree impossible by any other means.

Thus it becomes a case of 'creating before carousal': ' building before belligerency': 'gardening before golf' and 'satisfaction before satiety': and *sanity* above all.

It cannot be over-stressed, for survival – for intelligent survival and longevity, that there must be some return by man to the natural environment, the elements, in a word, the simple life of the country or the sea-shore.

CHAPTER TWENTY

It is for every man to work this out according to his own interest, capacities, finance and future planning. *But: something should be done!*

Summary of Chapter Twenty

The modern large city carries within itself many lethal conditions.

The solution to this problem is to leave the city where one's livelihood may compel one to reside, as often as possible.

The secret of healthy longevity will be found under rural conditions if it is ever to be found at all. Therefore, aim at a country house, no matter how modest. It is even better to design and build the domicile with one's own hands, or at least, as much as is reasonably possible.

A return to horticulture, growing one's own vegetables and fruits, perhaps some hens, can rest the brain, stimulate the mind, satisfy the primitive needs now being stifled in the large city, and not only advance longevity to a remarkable degree, but regenerate the whole organism – the psyche and the physical, for the return to the unavoidable city environment.

Chapter Twenty One

In conclusion, and to repeat.

Given our initial inheritance, physically and mentally, which we must accept although we can build up on both, we are finally, ultimately, and irrevocably, what we eat, drink and breathe.

Even the mind, and its processes, is dependent upon our physical state, since a sick body implies a sick mind somewhere, hence the dictum –

Only THE FIT ARE FEARLESS

Every unfit, diseased, even merely weak cell in our bodies causes an unfavourable reaction, through the nervous system, in our mind processes. Although when we view some brilliant minds this fact may not be obvious, it is nevertheless true.

The Greeks, some two thousand odd years ago realised this, hence their devotion to the gymnasium (the Greek word for Athleticism) and the evolvement of the various Games, of which the Olympic Games are the best known.

Also the coining of the adage – *Mens sana in corpore sano* – (a sound mind in a sound body) indicating that the Ancients knew the one without the other was impossible in fact.

It should be accepted: we can control our destiny: our level of health and fitness: our use value in the world: and our longevity, much more than the unfit, or the unthinking, can ever believe possible.

CHAPTER TWENTY ONE

Courage: endurance: zest: these are not mental states to be conjured up at will, but are the mental expression of physical states.

Just as we may state – 'Only the Fit are Fearless', so we must postulate, by contrary. 'The Unfit, by virtue of their condition, must be fearful.'

It is the customary physical unfitness: the lack of muscular tone: the low level of organ efficiency that is reflected in the minds of most of the world's countless millions.

It may yet be recognised that these factors, not the developed philosophies, ideologies, and religions, are the basic cause of the many fears, the feelings of insecurity, that so universally beset mankind.

All jealousy, envy, and feelings of inferiority generally, arise in the minds of the unfit. It is true, fitness implies action, competition and the concept of success, but never, fundamentally, on the elimination, much less the extermination, of the other.

Fitness does not need racialism, nationalism, religions, or ideologies of any kind to bolster it.

Fitness rests in itself, since the fit feel and recognise that they can wrest from life what is essential to their needs, and not necessarily at the expense of or exploitation of others.

Fitness, above all, pays dividends as no other investment really can.

Fitness does not, and never did, imply impecuniosity. All the world's men, noted for their high level of fitness, made ample money for their needs. None ever died impoverished.

Therefore: Be Fit! Be Healthy! Be rich in the world's goods: in all that this life can offer: it is for YOU to find, and to have, the means to seize them.

If you have absorbed this message then we can say, in all sincerity –

Jacta elea est: (The die has been cast)

'I am now committed'.

Some Conclusions

APPENDIX ONE: mostly philosophic

Life is not looking (being a spectator), or owning, it is 'living'. Living is not only getting and gaining, but 'doing'. Doing is not always doing something because it 'pays', but because it brings well-being to oneself, perhaps happiness to others. 'Doing' suggests a fuller life.

A fuller life means we are living the 'Good Life'.

The Good Life is when we leave the world a little better than we found it; that we have contributed, not just taken.

A contribution is made when we assist positively. A positive contribution can only be truly made when we use the benefit of our education, experience, money and the individualisation of ourselves in the service of others. That we live not just for ourselves.

We cannot live, and will not want to live, only for ourselves when we retain fitness, good-health and a forward-looking philosophy.

A forward-looking life, even at 80, is a life where you are planning ahead for activity, work trips.

Activity and work mean you never completely retire.

Retirement, when accepted fully, is the beginning of the end.

The end comes when the spirit gives up.

The spirit gives up when it is realised we have seen the lot: savoured the lot: done all, or most things, been most places:

experienced most things. With most men the spirit is prematurely broken down and gives up because of disappointment: disillusionment: or the realisation of an incurable disease. Or from the sheer boredom of living a useless life. Rejuvenation of the body, then, is firstly of the spirit.

The spirit is the 'life-spirit'. And the life-spirit in us exists just as we feel a vital interest in living. A vital interest in living will not permit us to feel content to sit all day, and every day, in a counting-house counting.

The life-spirit in us will count it as lost if we haven't gained the respect of our fellows. and the love of women and children.

These, then, are the ultimates, since money, alone, cannot buy them, although it can be helpful.

Being the ultimates they are worth repeating: Firstly, the respect of our fellow-man. Not just the admiration, nor the fear, but the respect. After all, what else can be as valuable, between men.

Then, there is the love of women, for ourselves, not just what we represent, or stand in front of: Women can be bought, but holding their affection and loyalty requires something more than success or money.

The affection of little children is something entirely unique, since children have little or no comprehension of the factors that can influence adults. You just have to be the right sort of person to gain the trust and affection (as distinct from cupboard love) of little children.

The acquirement of wealth does not prevent a man gaining the respect of others. Indeed, where there has been unusual success there can be marked respect. It is when the methods used to acquire wealth have been dubious that the rich lose the respect of honest men.

Money of itself cannot buy health. It can buy the essential food, make possible exercise and rest periods, trips and holidays that regenerate the spirit.

Without some money it is impossible to live at all in a civilized community.

With insufficient money it is impossible to live fully. With ample money it is possible to help others to live more fully.

Money spent on helping and teaching others to live more fully and healthily is better than money spent in endowing hospitals, no matter how necessary such hospitals may be.

How foolish, then, not to exert oneself to find the means, and to use the means, that can mean we live more fully, healthily, and as long in years as we want to live. To live until only the husk of life is left: until we have sucked the orange of life dry.

All things are possible: But it is we who must find the means: do the essential work, and consider the means worthwhile. It can be so.

APPENDIX TWO 'IF' (with apologies to Rudyard Kipling)

If you do not cut down your *refined* starches and sugars to the absolute minimum, or better, exclude them totally from your dietary: if you do not keep your intake of animal fats e.g., butter, lard, dripping, and the like, and the foods cooked in, or with them – to the absolute minimum: if you do not carefully watch the effect of alcohol on your liver: if you do not completely abandon the use of Nicotine (tobacco) in any form as an addiction with no useful or positive advantage: if you fail to realise the ultimate effect on your longevity, and the present effect on your physical and sexual abilities, of being over-weight: if you cannot accept the proposition that one stone (14Ib.) over-weight can mean five to ten years off your life expectancy, all other factors being satisfied: if you now realise that a diet of natural foods, your hunger controlled and naturally satisfied, as it can be: your weight factor cared for, even if you do not exercise, you still may live to an advanced age:

that whilst you do remain alive your brain can function efficiently, and your mind improve with each year and each decade: if you can accept, all these concepts and precepts and act in accordance with them, at least you will never become one of those slowly perambulating, hardly animated human parodies that we see so often and described as being 'elderly'.

If we add intelligent and consistent exercise to the point of sweating, and on most days, we can find we remain a fully-functioning, 'alive', active masculine animal, enjoying living even more than is the prerogative of the young, since we can now have the wisdom: the absence of worries: the understanding, and above all – the absence of phobias, tensions and breakdowns, and which every year besets the young more and more.

Let us state it, and accept it: This life is NOT for the young – but for the fit, healthy, travelled, and well-informed older man, who has, as he will have – retained his zest, capacities and functions, as he well might: or, as we now know – HE CAN!

APPENDIX THREE: a recapitulation of the book in axiomatic form

1. Adequate in quality nutriment
1. An absolute minimum of nutriment consistent with living
2. Complete bowel elimination
3. Sufficient exercise but no excess
4. Natural resistance to orthodoxy in every form
5. Capacity to ignore customary, even so-called scientific, pronouncements as to the life-span
6. An understanding of time and Relativity
7. An instinctive avoidance of medication
8. A resistance to alcohol: this need not necessarily imply total

prohibition but definitely an intake within the capacity of the organism to deal with its toxic effects. The normal toxic effects may well be off-set by the psychological value
9. A total avoidance of Nicotine and all other drugs
10. A resistance to the idea that the organism is failing: and the acceptance of the contrary notion that where the spirit is willing the body will provide the means
11. The falling back on the instinctive intelligence in all matters dealing with '11'. This means a denial of the idea that one is covered or dominated by what is found to be true of the norm
12. The everlasting – until it no longer is desired, rebirth of interests: this involves a zest for life and an understanding of the principles of regeneration; and the practice thereof:
13. The complete ejection from the mind of all that has been placed in it – and a re-education or revaluation of all relevant matters
14. An adoption of the notion of complete sovereignty as to oneself: this involves the acceptance in some degree of the idea of Existentialism
15. The recognition of the governing of life by dualism: the recognition of the part of determination and acceptance as basic
16. The understanding of what is meant by true intellectualism as distinct from academics
17. The recognition that there are no 'proofs' for anyone other than those demonstrated in action, i.e., 'living'.
18. That logic is relative not absolute.
19. That there is no other Principle but the Life Principle: all else is variable.
20. That the 'understanding' is in us – never to be discovered outside of us: this means that the search must be 'within'
21. That nothing at all – nothing! must be accepted as absolute or fixed: that all is in a state of flux

22. That these matters as they apply to the concept of the Universe its origins: meaning: etc. can be understood and captured through the mystical sense: but this sense can only be based in scientific knowledge – but the sense can outdistance the knowledge. Without this sense all scientific knowledge must be finite.
23. That because any other individual may not have as full a realisation as perhaps another does not mean in any way the limitations that some believe and impose.

APPENDIX FOUR: *suggestions for dietary*

It must be accepted that different countries and customs, as different climates, have greatly influenced the dietary habits of peoples. However, there is no doubt or question at all that those peoples, such as the Hunzas, who live on what is best termed, 'Nature's Foods', that is – foods as found naturally growing, and before such foods have been refined and factorised, such peoples tend to live healthily and to a degree of longevity not known in the Western World, or in those countries with a deficient dietary.

The lists as appended are not arbitrary and should be used as a guide only. However, if you are over 40, or over-weight at any age, or take little or no vigorous exercise, you are well-advised to confine your food intake to the foods set out in Column 1.

If you are under 40, not over-weight, and especially if you live a vigorous life as to work or exercise, your dietary problems are solved in both Columns 1 and 2.

If you are over 70 years of age, no matter how you live, or exercise, you will be wise to confine your foods to those listed in Column 1

Column 3 contains the list of foods better considered as 'banned', although the occasional use will be in no way detrimental to health. It

SOME CONCLUSIONS

is the habitual use of foods not considered suitable that causes Nature to punish by unfitness, obesity, cancers, heart and arterial diseases, etc.

However, the wise will find no sacrifices are felt or made once the habit of eating the foods listed in Column 3 abandoned. Indeed, a greater relish will be enjoyed and a more true appetite experienced. Hunger is controllable, and should be (See Table on pages 172 and 175)

These suggestions are by no means meant to be a complete guide or a complete list. The approach must be one of common sense, and not appetite or prejudice. If the food cannot be recognised as an article in Nature, or basically so, it should be suspect as good food. It is the life-principle in our food that, absorbed by our system, provides us with the only life-force we can function on, and survive. Hence 'live' foods lead to life: 'Dead' foods lead to the grave. Definitely, we are, and can be –

'ONLY WHAT WE EAT'

SOME CONCLUSIONS

Column 1	Column 2	Column 3
Suitable for all persons. Any age: any occupation	Suitable for the younger person or those who exercise above average	Foods best banned from the dietary entirely
All Vegetables, eaten raw in Salads, or lightly steamed or baked. In the case of Potatoes, best French-fried (chipped) in oil, or baked in jackets. All Fruits in season: best eaten ripe and uncooked, in toto or in salads: Ripe bananas especially good since they replace bread. All Meats, other than Pork: (Bacon an exception). All poultry. All sea-foods. Bacon. Eggs, fresh, raw or lightly cooked. Cheese – mild. Milk – only as a flavouring in tea and coffee. Rolled Oatmeal: (raw or lightly cooked). Dried Fruits, i.e., Raisins, Prunes, etc. Nuts: softer kernels best, i.e., walnuts. Olive Oil or other vegetable cooking oils.	Ham. Cheeses: tasty varieties. *Wholemeal*, Breads, Scones, Buns, Biscuits, Cakes. Fruit Cakes. Puddings. Custard. Ice-cream. Canned Fruit, jams, various 'spreads' such as Vegemite. Honey. Rice and other cereals used in cooking and soups. Confectionery – Chocolate (on occasion). Spaghetti and Macaroni. Sauces and Pickles. Thick Soups, using meat, vegetables, barley, etc. Fluids as per Column 1.	Refined Flour (white) and all its products. e.g., biscuits, breads, scones, etc. Pastry and Pastries. Refined Sugar (white) and its overuse in cooking and confectionery. All animal fat, e.g., butter, cream, lard, dripping. (N.B. Margarine is neither advised or necessary.) All packeted and pre-cooked breakfast foods and cereals. Mashed potato. All vegetables that have been steeped in water, when cooked and the water thrown away. Pepper and Mustard.

Column 1	Column 2	Column 3
Suitable for all persons. Any age: any occupation	Suitable for the younger person or those who exercise above average	Foods best banned from the dietary entirely
Note here: to bring down the weight breakfast can be dispensed with: at best two or three pieces of ripe fruit, or two or three cups of tea or coffee. *Fluids*: Water, at any time. Fruit juices, fresh or canned. Tea: Coffee, but *never with*, or after meals, always *before* eating, and then limited to twice daily. Incidentally: no morning or afternoon-teas, or suppers. Alcohol: in moderation. Wine permitted with a meal, or after food has been taken.	If exercising hard, e.g., a fully trained middle-distance runner, oarsman, and the like, a Vit B Complex tablet and one Vit C 500 m.g. tablet may be added to the diet, as also Wheat Germ can be used. It is important to note that Column 1 is to be considered the main source of bodily nutriment. Column 2 merely additional items used in certain circumstances.	It is not proved that common salt is either essential or other than harmful. Certainly its use should be kept to the very minimum. Salt is NOT necessary in conservative cooking. All colouring matters and flavourings especially those known to have a coal-tar basis (cancer promoting).

NOTES ON YOUR FITNESS

NOTES ON YOUR FITNESS

Also by the same author, the classic revival of

ATHLETICS: HOW TO BECOME A CHAMPION

Is now available on www.amazon.com

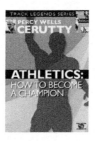

Coming soon:

MIDDLE DISTANCE RUNNING

BY PERCY WELLS CERUTTY

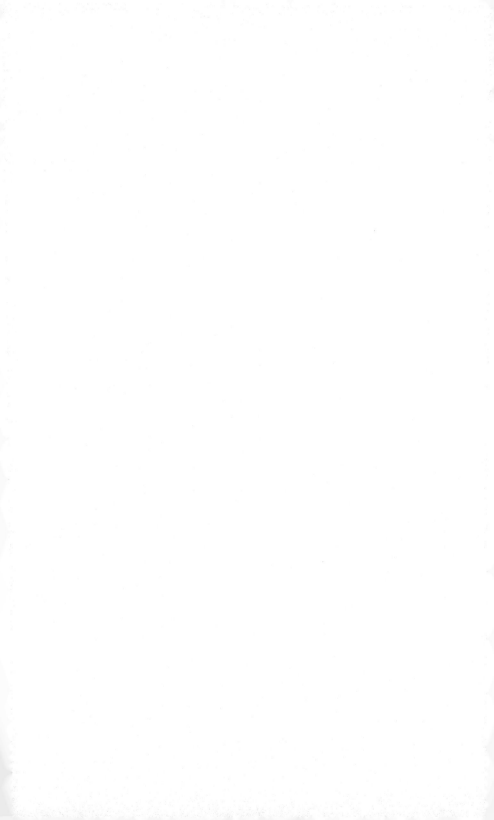